Praise for *The Dark Side of the Mind*

'Enthralling and terrifying. *The Dark Side of the Mind* is a chilling glimpse into a world of miscreants, monsters and the misunderstood.'
– Professor Dame Sue Black, author of *Sunday Times* bestseller *All That Remains*

'Kerry Daynes delves into the minds of psychopaths in a fascinating memoir.'
– Katya Edwards, *Daily Mail*

'Daynes offers fascinating insights into what makes criminals tick and how they might be more effectively treated. Her book is funny, wise and thoroughly gripping.'
– Jake Kerridge, writer and critic

'Grimly fascinating – a timely and gripping exploration of mental health issues in the criminal justice system from an author intimately acquainted with its dark heart.'
– Harriet Tyce, author of *Blood Orange*

THE DARK SIDE OF THE MIND

True Stories From My Life
As A Forensic Psychologist

Kerry Daynes

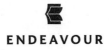

ENDEAVOUR

An Hachette UK Company
www.hachette.co.uk

First published in Great Britain in 2019 by Endeavour, an imprint of
Octopus Publishing Group Ltd
Carmelite House
50 Victoria Embankment
London EC4Y 0DZ
www.octopusbooks.co.uk

This edition published in 2020

ISBN 978-1-78840-217-0

A CIP catalogue record for this book is available from the British
Library.

Printed and bound in Great Britain

10 9 8 7

CONTENTS

Author's Note   vii
Prologue   1

Chapter 1: Here Be Monsters   11
Chapter 2: Big Boys Don't Cry   31
Chapter 3: The Blame Game   47
Chapter 4: Faking It   75
Chapter 5: Witchdoctors and Brainwashers   101
Chapter 6: Power Plays   129
Chapter 7: Insults and Injuries   159
Chapter 8: A Man's World   185
Chapter 9: The Case of the Missing Finger   219
Chapter 10: Safe and Sound   237
Chapter 11: The Sum of Our Parts   259

Epilogue   281

Interview with the Author   289
Reading Group Questions   299

Notes and Further Reading   303
Acknowledgements   310
About the Author   312

To Mum, Dad and Big Sis

Author's Note

The stories you read here are based on my recollections, experiences and life as a forensic psychologist. Names and certain identifying details have been changed to protect the privacy of the innocent, and the bang-to-rights guilty. And, moreover, to protect myself. I spend enough time in court as it is.

If thou gaze long into an abyss,
the abyss will also gaze into thee.
Friedrich Nietzsche

Prologue

Sometimes you help your patients see things more clearly, sometimes they help you.

Maurice was in his 80s, his long, thin frame so twisted with arthritis that from a distance he looked like a gnarled old hawthorn tree. One that was dressed up like Simon Cowell, all high-waisted trousers and tight white T-shirts. He had a glass eye too, giving him an off-centre gaze that added to his general asymmetry.

He wasn't on my caseload, but was one of the long-term residents at a hospital secure unit where I'd recently started a new job as a soon-to-be-qualified psychologist. The hospital was on the edge of a sprawling and impoverished council estate on the outskirts of a depressed northern town – you could say it was gritty.

Unless you've personally been detained in a secure unit under the Mental Health Act, it can be hard to understand the difference between these places and plain old prison. The two settings treat their guests very differently. In the prison service the approach is ordered and dominated by the need to provide security and protection for the public. In secure hospitals, such as this one, the approach is to have as few restrictions as possible – to be more collaborative; not only containing, but actively caring. Like prisoners, the people here aren't at liberty; they are considered to pose a danger to themselves or, more likely, to others. But because many of these environments are divided into smaller, almost homely, units with shared communal living areas, it's not that unusual to find members of staff eating lunch alongside their patients.

So it was that I would find myself on most Tuesdays and Thursdays popping over to the small annexe where Maurice lived, to spend my lunch break with the occupants of Milton Ward.

Maurice's psychiatric reports made repeated mention of his suffering from a 'sexual sadism disorder'. The irony of the word 'suffering' wasn't lost on me. Sexual sadists experience intense sexual thrills in response to the pain, humiliation, distress or general torment of another living thing. This is not to be confused with some experimental spanking or even the more toe-curlingly creative antics mutually entered into by latex-clad submissives and dominants. Sexual sadism is only considered a disorder – and there is a disorder for pretty much everything – if the individual acts on their urges with someone non-consenting. Which raises the question: who is really suffering here?

For Maurice, this meant that he liked to lurk in isolated spots and whip out what should have been his private parts at unsuspecting girls and women. The shock and horror on their faces was a source of exquisite personal and sexual pleasure for him. His penchant for this cheapest of thrills had briefly landed him in prison as a young man, but unsurprisingly this didn't curb him. After his release he graduated to the point at which two women were found dead in his home, each with multiple stab wounds of varying depths, predominantly centred around their breasts. The precise explorations of a torturer. Now an established resident at the secure unit, Maurice wasn't going anywhere. Ever.

One Tuesday, while I was having my lunch at the annexe – soup and a bread roll – Maurice approached me from behind and in the blink, quite literally, of an eye, popped his ocular prosthesis straight out of his face and into my Heinz Cream of Tomato. Before I could process what was happening, I was covered in blood-red spatters and my soup was gazing back at me.

Still somewhat green around the edges at 24, I momentarily lost self-control and gave Maurice exactly the reaction he was hoping for. I shrieked, physically leapt out of my seat, my Celtic complexion turning an even whiter shade of pale. Who wouldn't balk when faced with an eyeball in their soup?

I'd been aware of Maurice's glass eye beforehand, but it turns out that when you see one doing backstroke in your soup your brain instinctively tells you it's an actual eyeball. A jellied part of someone else's body.

The rational explanation – that it's really nothing more than a giant marble – kicks in a while later, once you've screamed the place down.

I got a quick look at his face – a sunken crevice where his eyeball had been, the healthy eye looking intently at me, studying my reaction – and caught a hint of a smirk as he was ushered off by a male nurse. I began to kick myself. This old man had just got the better of me.

This was an example of 'offence paralleling' – when a person behaves in a pattern that resembles or serves the same function as his criminal behaviour. For Maurice, the sense of mastery at producing fear and disgust on the face of the nearest woman, via the sudden exposure of this particular body part, was as good as it was going to get in the limiting confines of the hospital environment.

I felt enormous embarrassment for walking into Maurice's trap that day. But the encounter helped me understand a great deal about the profession I had chosen to enter. Because how do you solve a problem like Maurice? The conundrum of this man, and the way I reacted to him, is the challenge at the heart of the forensic psychology I practise every day.

Dealing with Maurice might seem obvious to some – surely you just take away the false eyeball? But I'm not the sadist in this story. It's not my remit or desire to punish or humiliate the people I work with. And simply taking it away wouldn't address the root problem – his need to shock and the sexual gratification he took from it. If we removed the glass eyeball, his drives would find another way to manifest themselves. And let's not forget that removing a person's body parts, even prosthetic ones, tends to raise some pretty awkward human rights questions.

There will be those who argue that eating lunch in the same room as Maurice was asking for trouble. Who in their right mind has lunch with a convicted sex offender and doesn't expect to catch his eye, figuratively at least? But this puts the onus on the victim (in this case, me) to alter my behaviour – to find somewhere else to eat my lunch. And it's my job to help men like Maurice change *their* behaviour. Besides, starving his problem of the oxygen it needs (for Maurice, simply access to women) doesn't necessarily kill it. It can just make it more desperate to survive.

Sticks or stones may break my bones, but an eye in my lunch is, at worst, nothing more than a choking hazard. As I was reminded the hard way on that day, an effective approach to extinguishing any kind of unpleasant behaviour in this environment, where it is safe to do so, is simply to ignore it. Any parent of toddlers can verify this – it's the most basic of behaviourist techniques. (Behaviourists are firmly on one side of the nature vs. nurture debate. They assert that we're all born blank slates and only do anything because we have learned it from other people, and then persist with this behaviour depending upon the degree to which it is rewarded or punished.) And as any parent of toddlers will also confirm, not providing the sought-after reaction to a behaviour is often one of the hardest approaches to implement.

As Maurice shuffled off and my heart began to beat a little slower, I realized that if I was going to make it in this career – if I was ever going to find the best solutions to the problems that my patients present – I needed to learn to override my own emotional responses. I needed to manage my own healthy, automatic revulsion at such disturbing behaviour and carry on regardless.

I'd have to push the eyeball to one side, and keep drinking the soup.

*

Lunch with Maurice was only one of the many extraordinary experiences I've had in my 20 years as a forensic psychologist. I've worked with some of society's most troubled and troubling offenders, in prisons, hospitals, courts and police stations, in neighbourhoods and communities just like yours. Experiences which have changed me and the way I see the world indelibly.

I'm sometimes referred to as a criminal psychologist, which sounds like I'm on the Mafia payroll. In truth I have very little to do with criminology (the study of crime trends and crime prevention). Some other things I don't do include detective work (no wrestling suspects to the ground) and pathology (no chopping up dead bodies – although a serial killer once showed me how to dismember a turkey).

All crimes are committed by – and happen to – people. Forensic psychology is about them.

A large part of my job is trying to reduce reoffending among those who have committed crimes, with the ultimate aim of making society a safer place. To do this, I apply the scientific methods of psychology to try to understand the mental processes behind the criminal act. The challenge for psychologists is then to attempt to take steps to help the person change their behaviour, and begin their new life as a fully reformed, law-abiding citizen. This is the holy grail. More frequently, however, I advise others on the safe and appropriate response to a kaleidoscope of extreme behaviour, anything from fire setting to child killing. My evaluations, assessments and testimonies help inform the decisions of judges and juries, parole boards, police and mental health teams. Decisions that have the power to profoundly affect people's lives.

It's a role that's wedged awkwardly between the criminal justice and mental health systems. These overburdened and innately flawed institutions make a curmudgeonly couple, both of them old and confused, like the grandparents in Roald Dahl's *Charlie and the Chocolate Factory*, forced to share a bed they are too slow and seized up to get out of.

I prefer to call the people I work with 'clients'. It might sound irritatingly politically correct, more like I am a nail technician than a forensic psychologist, but I use this term as a respectful umbrella for the wide variety of people I come into contact with. It's an inescapable fact that most of my clients are men, but they are also occasionally women. I work with victims as well as offenders. Often it transpires that my clients have, at some point in their lives, been both.

*

People have always been morbidly enthralled by crime and criminals – from Jack the Ripper theories to the controversial conviction of Steven Avery – especially those who go against the most sacred values of society and commit the brutally violent and sexual crimes that are so incomprehensible to us all. For those of us who play by the rule book, few things are more fascinating, and more rankling, than those who choose to tear it apart. It's perhaps no surprise then that our news and entertainment channels brim with stories from the wrong side of the law – it's hard to imagine our thirst for it ever being slaked.

But so often these stories focus on what is really only a small chapter in the bigger tale. They tell us about the crime that's been committed, the subsequent investigation through to the trial, the conviction and the sentencing of the guilty person. What happens afterwards is rarely talked about, as if the criminal, and all the consequences of their actions, have disappeared in a puff of smoke. But life doesn't end for that person, or their families or their victims. They have to learn to live with it, forever. A psychologist can join the story at any stage, but it is very often at the point at which the court proceedings have concluded, after the media and public interest wanes, that we become key characters in the narrative.

The stories I've chosen to tell here are the ones you probably won't read about in the papers. They focus on the everyday work of being a forensic psychologist, in all its frustrating, conflicting and just occasionally life-affirming reality.

I've included these particular stories for many reasons – some are heartbreaking, others are enraging, some are just plain weird. What connects them is my personal sense of having been affected by them. That, and the insight they give us into the extremes of our shared human condition.

The question I am asked perhaps more than any other, whether it's by a taxi driver with whom I'm passing the time of day or a judge who wants my professional opinion, is: What the hell is wrong with these people? The words may be more or less formal, but everyone really wants to know the same thing. What is so wrong with someone that he or she commits a serious crime? Because once we know what's wrong with someone, we can fix them, right? Or confine them, out of harm's way. It took me a long time – too long – to realize that we're all asking the wrong question.

CHAPTER 1
HERE BE MONSTERS

*The degree of civilization in a society
can be judged by entering its prisons.*
Fyodor Dostoevsky

When I tell people I'm a forensic psychologist they usually express surprise and start mentally fumbling around for the least offensive way to tell me that I don't look how a forensic psychologist should (for most people the acceptable archetype still seems to be Cracker, the world-weary alcoholic and gambling-addicted loose cannon, played by Robbie Coltrane in the 1990s TV series). They'll often say I'm too petite or delicate. Sometimes they do a sort of awkward hourglass movement with their hands. What they are keenly observing, but terribly articulating, is that I am a woman.

In fact, most of the forensic psychologists I know are women. Women make up 73 per cent of the British Psychological Society (the professional body for practising psychologists in the United Kingdom), and a whopping 80 per cent of its forensic division. Why so many X chromosomes? I can't speak for the other

2,035 of us, but psychology appealed to me because it promised a way of making sense of things, models and theories for understanding an otherwise overwhelming world. There seemed a promise of safety and security in having that user manual. That, and the fact that it is endlessly fascinating; your own glimpse into the private events of someone else's mind. It was seductive to the young me.

If I am honest with myself, I was also swayed by a law student whose name I'll never forget: Stephen P English. My decision to also take a law option as part of my psychology degree at Sheffield University was made – as all the best freshers' week decisions are – under the influence of hormones and cheap cider. I took the law subsidiary purely and simply so that I could gaze at his beautiful head from the back of the lecture hall, imagining what the P stood for. Perfection? Pectorals? Perhaps.

It was pure accident that I found myself enjoying law. So forensic psychology – forensic is Latin for *of the forum*, or law courts – seemed like a sensible career choice. Happy endings being the stuff of fairy tales, I never actually plucked up the courage to talk to Stephen P English and ended up dating an older PhD student throughout my university years instead. He had long dark hair, chain smoked roll-ups and wore a full-length Driza-Bone waxed coat. When it was raining, which in Sheffield was always, he wore a matching wide-brimmed hat. He'd stride into the student union bar like Clint Eastwood into a saloon. When he was drunk, or stoned – which was also always – he would get maudlin and declare 'there's no justice, it's just us'. I had no idea what he was talking about and, I suspect, neither did he.

*

As a young girl I often spent Saturday nights at my gran's house, watching spaghetti westerns on her black and white television. She was a classic Irish-Catholic matriarch, who somehow always managed to look at least 50 years older than she was: tight perm, blue rinse, crimplene dresses and a plastic rain cap. She worked in a yoghurt factory in Manchester, and part of the uniform was green wellies, so the whole family had green yoghurt-factory wellies. We'd sit and watch cowboy films or anything with John Wayne in. Gran's favourite was *The Quiet Man*. I liked it too because Maureen O'Hara was the only film star I'd ever seen with red hair, and this was long before being ginger was fashionable. It would just be my gran and me and Joey, my Great-Uncle John's yellow canary. People who did bad things – the 'badjuns' as my gran called them when they came on screen – seemed reassuringly different to me, from another planet even.

The films I watched with my gran instilled in me a clear-cut notion of good versus evil, assuming the inevitable triumph of the virtuous, which the otherwise sheer uneventfulness of my childhood reinforced. I was fortunate to have a comfortable and unremarkable upbringing, crime simply didn't affect me, my family or anyone I knew at that time. In my early teens the closest I came to real-life badjuns were the warnings of flashers in the park I heard from girls at school, or the occasional news of a neighbour being burgled. It was only the late-night, slurred conversations about law and order I had at university that prompted a growing awareness of and interest in the big crime stories of the day.

*

During the years I was at university – 1992 to 1995 – law and order had become a touchstone of the political agenda. In February 1993, two-year-old James Bulger was tortured and murdered by Robert Thompson and Jon Venables. The nation watched CCTV footage of Jamie being led away from the New Strand shopping centre, hand-in-hand with one of his killers, and was united in its horror and fury. As tabloid headlines went full throttle (there was no tolerance here, not even for ten-year-old killers, especially for ten-year-old killers), both main political parties saw their chance to win votes by demonstrating a hard line on crime.

Despite the hen's-teeth rarity of primary school children who kill, shadow Home Secretary Tony Blair was quick to declare the case symbolic of the 'sleeping' moral conscience of the country under Tory rule, while simultaneously launching Labour's 'tough on crime, tough on the causes of crime' policy. Days after the arrest of James's killers, John Major, then Prime Minister, reciprocated with a call for society 'to condemn a little more and understand a little less'. It was the start of a mushrooming in prisoner numbers that would see them more than double throughout my career, from around 44,000 when I started my studies in 1992 to almost 87,000 in 2018.

Prison is the largest employer of forensic psychologists in the UK, so I knew early on I'd need to get some work experience inside *inside*. Prison psychologists run various offending-behaviour programmes that promise to transform the thinking of offenders and reduce their risk of reoffending upon release. This was part of the tough and supposedly effective stance on criminality the public had bought into – quite literally, as millions of pounds of taxpayers' money had just begun to be poured into running these programmes. For me, prison wasn't only a punishment or deterrent but a place to rehabilitate and reform; I was ready to roll my sleeves up and get stuck in. I'd already volunteered on a victim and offender mediation programme (mostly an exercise in stopping the two parties from coming to blows) and had trained as an appropriate adult, sitting in on police station interviews with vulnerable suspects – people who've ended up in trouble and are young, have learning difficulties or mental health problems. What I didn't realize at the time was that I might have benefited from an appropriate adult myself.

HMP Manchester, rebranded from Strangeways after the riots, was the first prison I set foot in, albeit only briefly. I had just turned 20. I'd managed to arrange a quick careers talk from the prison psychologist, followed by a tour of E and F wings, a mixture of cells and education rooms. A prison officer, who made no effort to disguise the fact that he'd drawn the short straw in showing me the sights, rushed me around the 'twos' (the first-floor landing) of E wing, all shiny painted brickwork and blue metal doors and railings. HMP Manchester has very little natural light and had an aroma not unlike the student flats I lived in. I scuttled along behind my escort, smiling at the inmates as I passed by their cells – men in identikit grey sweatshirts, milling in and out of identikit magnolia spaces. When the entire place erupted in high shrieks of 'Meow!', echoing like a vocal Mexican wave around the Victorian vaults, I asked him why they were making cat noises. He just rolled his eyes. (In case you haven't guessed, it was to alert fellow prisoners that some pussy had arrived.)

*

The atmosphere at HMP Wakefield was considerably less bouncy.

It was summer 1996, I was a year out of university, the Spice Girls were number one and I really wanted to be a forensic psychologist. I had written to all the prisons on the northern circuit, volunteering my services. Wakefield – known affectionately to its residents as the armpit of Yorkshire – was the only place that replied. They had a project for me. There was no pay, but I didn't care. I was going to single-handedly reduce the crime rate, and here was an opportunity to put some real experience on my CV. Besides, I had £36 a week income support, and if I took the employment training course they were pushing at the Job Centre, I'd get an *extra tenner* on top of that. I bought myself a new suit from C&A and found a grotty flat-share above a Chinese takeaway – ladies and gentlemen, I had arrived.

The average prisoner at HMP Wakefield was older than the boisterous bunch at Strangeways and in for the long haul. They couldn't be bothered to shout at you in here and largely wouldn't have dared – the level of institutional control ran too deep. We're talking category A and B prisoners, the ones you really don't want to escape. (Category A prisoners require maximum security because their escape would be highly dangerous for the public or national security. B-listers are slightly less risky, but you still don't want to make it easy for them to arrange their own release.) Sex offenders made up around 10 per cent of the UK's overall prison population at that time, but still constituted the vast majority of Wakefield's inmates, many of them the most high-profile and publicly despised offenders. It's for this reason that journalists are obsessed with the place; it is still widely referred to in the media as Monster Mansion.

Monsters terrified me when I was a child. My dad let me stay up late one night to watch *Creature from the Black Lagoon* on television (I'm a child of the 1970s, all my cultural references are from television). My mum worked nights at a psychiatric hospital, so she wasn't there to point out what a terrible idea it was. I don't know why he thought I'd enjoy it, I'd already been taken out of *ET* during the first ten minutes of the screening because I was scared of a small waddling alien. I got through about three minutes of *Black Lagoon* before terror set in, the moment when a scaly webbed hand, attached to an unseen body, emerges from the water and then slowly slips back, trailing claw marks in the sand. Somehow it was more horrifying to me that you didn't know what was attached to that claw, than to see the actual creature. Perhaps in those first few minutes of a 1950s horror movie I had begun to suspect that dangerous things aren't always in plain sight.

*

There has been a prison at Wakefield since the 16th century, but most of the existing buildings are Victorian-era; long, multi-level galleries of cells leading off in different directions from a central hub, like a broken clock-face (they are doing time, after all). Prisons with radial designs like this were inspired by the 'panopticon' theories of the 18th-century English philosopher, Jeremy Bentham. His thinking was that, in this fan-like layout, every cell could be easily seen by a single watchman in the centre. Inmates would feel the weight of constant potential surveillance, and so modify their behaviour accordingly. In practice, of course, everyone knows that it is impossible to watch everybody at all times, and if you want to get up to no good you just choose an opportune moment in your cell. When I was working there, it wasn't unusual for the occasional dead pigeon to spiral down from the cell windows on the outside wall of A wing. Inmates fed them through holes that had been broken out over the years. Then – if they were so inclined – they broke their necks and sent the unfortunate birds plummeting, preferably just at the moment a member of staff was walking by underneath.

The psychology team at Wakefield wanted me to do the leg work on a research project, interviewing all of the prisoners who had both sexually assaulted and killed women. I was to find out how the assault had escalated and what might have turned a rapist into a murderer. My task was to collect information that could later be analysed under a number of motivational types for sex offenders: were they compensating for sexual inadequacy, angry, seeking a sense of power and control, sadistic or opportunistic? The information I collected would be used to develop guidelines for women to use during a sexual assault. The idea being that in the throes of being physically and mentally overpowered by a rapist, a woman could quickly identify her attacker's motivational profile and somehow adjust her behaviour in order to avoid possibly being killed.

That this was considered a suitable project for a young female graduate with no training or experience is gobsmacking enough. But also that anyone thought it appropriate research in the first place, when it so clearly suggests responsibility for the severity of the attack lies with the victim and not the criminal who is viciously attacking her. I can imagine the eventual leaflet, something you might pick up at the doctor's surgery: 'Ladies! Don't let woeful ignorance get you murdered! We always recommend that you avoid getting yourself raped, but, if you do, just follow this handy cut-out-and-keep guide.'

During my first week, before my project began in earnest, I went through the standard induction given to all new non-uniformed staff joining the prison. It was a routine week of tours and talks, mostly mundane practicalities such as the location of the toilets, what to do in a fire drill and how to carry your keys (securely attached by a chain to your belt, preferably in a pouch, and with your palm obscuring the bit that slides into the lock if you are holding them within sight of an inmate). But throughout the week, whoever I was with and whatever I was being shown, I was told about the Wakefield Way. It was like a school motto, something everyone there seemed proud to stand by. But it wasn't about valour or courage in the face of adversity, it was more about a shared adherence to one simple premise: it was, I was repeatedly informed, 'them and us'.

What everyone seemed to agree on, and to actively perpetuate, was a state of pseudo-moral warfare. On one side the inmates: a force of evil to be reviled and subjugated. On the other, the prison officers: blessed and unquestionable. It was a setup that comfortingly reflected the simplistic notions of good guys and bad guys that I had grown up watching in the films with my gran. In reality it was by no means a peaceful arrangement, the opposite of what today is known as 'dynamic' or 'relational security', where everyone tries to get along. The bubbling tension between officers and prisoners was palpable and relationships were unpleasant. Just the week before I arrived a prison officer, going about his routine morning unlock, had been slashed by an inmate with a razor sellotaped to the end of a toothbrush.

To show enthusiasm for the rehabilitation of prisoners, or suggest they were anything other than irretrievable, a write-off, was to be entirely on the wrong side – a traitor. One prison officer earnestly warned me that the psychologists here were all deluded do-gooders. Oh, and lesbians.

Eager to embark on my career, I got to work on my project. I was given a list of surnames and prison numbers of the inmates whose convictions included not only the murder of a woman, but also rape or sexual assault of the victim. And I got a questionnaire, a list of pretty much every sexual and violent thing you can do to a woman. (Some of it, like eviscerating – pulling a person's insides out – I'd never even heard of, never mind the associated sexual practices.) I had to go through the list asking if they had done this or that, and if I got an affirmative answer, I had to then ask them how their victim had responded and explore what other possible reactions might have led to.

It was a very long questionnaire, each interview took over an hour and a half, and asking men, any men, but particularly these convicted prisoners, explicit questions was embarrassing to say the least. I knew I was blushing as I went through the list but I tried my conscientious best to be a 'psychologist first and a woman second' (a vague and confusing nugget of advice I'd received from a supervisor).

Some interviews were more difficult than others to get through. One man told me he'd bitten off a woman's nipple because he was enraged that she hadn't tried to fight him off while he raped her. Proof, in his mind, that she was enjoying his assault and was therefore a 'whore'. Research tells us that at least 70 per cent of rape victims freeze like this, and, were I to meet him in a professional capacity today, we'd have a full and frank discussion about his reasoning. But I didn't know how to react to it then. I instinctively raised my hand to protectively cover my own breast but caught it in time, put it back down, wrote down his answer and went on to the next question. Others deliberately *made* it difficult, asking me to explain what the clinical language of the questionnaire meant in more detail ('What does to digitally penetrate mean, miss?'). To those bored and sex-deprived inmates, my sessions must have seemed more like a free call to an adult chat line than serious research. I was being thrown in at the deep end and left to swim among the sharks.

At least I had a script with the inmates. Interactions with some of my colleagues weren't turning out to be any easier. In the second week of interviews, I went to the central office and asked the officer behind the desk – a cantankerous bellyacher of a man – for a rape alarm (as opposed to just one of the plain old personal alarms that staff were issued with). He turned to the other officers in the busy room and said, 'Aw, do you think you are going to get *raped* today? The little girl thinks she is going to get *raped* today lads.' Then he demanded I hand over my shoes if I wanted an alarm, as my conservative mid-heels were clearly going to whip the inmates into a sexual frenzy. I walked away, without the alarm but still with my shoes, my eyes beginning to burn. As soon as I was far enough away from any judgemental eyes, I burst into tears.

One of the many things I would like to tell the 21-year-old me about my time at Wakefield is to notice the warning signs that were waving at me like giant 'Golf Sale' placards on a busy high street. But my eagerness to do a good job eclipsed any creeping doubts I had. I was excited to be starting my career. To have shown what I wrongly thought of as weakness, or, worse, to have complained, could have meant an end to my time there.

After my first few weeks, a kinder prison officer took me to one side and quietly pointed out that the security routine I was going through each morning on my way in – when a male officer would run his hands up and down my entire body, ostensibly to check I hadn't brought my machete to work – wasn't actually happening to any of the other female staff. Or in fact any staff, other than me.

The sound of cascading pennies clanged in my ears. Today we'd call it sexual harassment at best. But I wasn't yet tuned in to the concept of misogyny, certainly not assertive enough to call it out. And this was Yorkshire in the 1990s, they still had strippers in the pub on Sunday afternoons. Hashtags hadn't even been invented yet, never mind #metoo. The next time someone tried to give me my morning once-over I just gritted my teeth and laughed them off, instincts telling me that to reveal a loss of humour over this wouldn't do me any favours.

Wakefield is home to the Prison Service College, a training centre separate from the prison, and for many the job was in the family, a kind of destiny that seemed to give some of them an enhanced sense of power and entitlement. When, in 2004, a report from Her Majesty's Chief Inspector of Prisons described HMP Wakefield as 'over-controlled' with some officers showing disrespect to inmates, I wasn't surprised.

A few of the younger officers in particular seemed to regard themselves as princes – the prison was their castle, and they had all the keys. Many of them also had deep tans, acquired at the local sunbed salon, not in Wakefield's sultry climate. They'd pop out for a quick blast on their lunch break, and come back a disconcerting two shades darker than when they left. All part of their preening rituals, trying to attract a mate on a night out. There were rumours that a group of them would go out drinking on the Golden Mile – Wakefield's main party strip – and bring girls back to the prison car park to have sex with them under the peripheral security cameras, so their colleagues on night shift could be entertained. Again when I read about these 'high times' years later in press reports, I wasn't surprised. In fact my only reaction was to question why, at the time, I never placed this on the same spectrum of dodgy behaviour as the prisoners I was interviewing.

*

Some of the officers started asking me out on dates. I would later learn there was a book running, taking bets on who would win the race to get me into bed. My arrival at this overwhelmingly male facility, where any kind of female had immediate novelty value, was causing a stir.

Co-favourite at 3:1, and the first to approach me, also happened to be the senior officer on C wing (there was a pecking order, even when it came to bedding the newbies): Prison Officer John Hall. He approached me while I was reading notes in the records room, where information about the inmates was held. Press clippings, disciplinary charges and adjudications, complaints and prison correspondence with family members, and just about anything else deemed relevant, were kept in here. Some of the files even contained crime scene pictures – these gruesome elements of an inmate's legal paperwork were confiscated from them if they were caught offering them to others as masturbation material or using them for bragging purposes.

This was before digitized records, so it was all kept in standard-issue manila folders, rows and rows of them along the entire far wall of this long thin room, each marked by hand with a prisoner's surname and number. Thanks to Wakefield's notorious alumni (Charles Bronson, IRA chief of staff Cathal Goulding, Jeremy

Bamber, Michael Sams and Colin Ireland had all signed the visitors' book) it was a cross between *Who's Who* and the Chamber of Horrors.

John Hall came in as I was reading Ireland's paperwork, reeling slightly at the nature of the file. Ireland had murdered five gay men and left their corpses in various macabre and undignified poses – a motif that was intended to send a message of contempt to the police and the media reporting the case. The file contained a clutch of letters from Ireland's fans, the likes of which I had never seen. Extreme, far-right homophobes had written to congratulate Ireland on his work, and the letters had been intercepted and found their way to his file, complete with their hand-drawn swastikas. I was looking at the letters and pondering, What the hell is wrong with these people?

There was nothing special about the way he asked me out. He walked past the records room, did a U-turn after he saw me sitting there, and came in and sat down next to me. Hall was – probably still is – a big, tall lump of a man, so I couldn't exactly pretend that I hadn't noticed him. He asked how I was settling in, did I need any help or someone to show me Wakefield, and, eventually, did I want to go out for a drink with him? I didn't. Politely, I said thank you but no. Then, because I felt I had to justify not wanting to go out on a date with this person, I said that someone else had already asked me out and I was considering it. They hadn't and I wasn't – but I'd said it out loud now.

The next officer to ask me out was a good few years older than me and not the kind of man I would have ever imagined myself being involved with. But I was lonely in Wakefield without my friends and family close by, and he was handsome – and persistent.

My time at Wakefield was coming to an end. The research I'd been working on had been quietly dropped, as numerous projects are. I had been redirected to more appropriate tasks, conducting a dull staff communication survey and doing admin for a treatment programme for sex offenders. But I still wasn't getting a pay cheque at Wakefield and so had been applying for paid positions at the same time. (Eventually I got a job as a trainee forensic psychologist in a secure hospital – my first real job. I'd be swapping prisoners for patients soon.)

When my new love interest told me he and his fellow officers had written a message to their inmates, 'Merry Christmas and may you get all that is coming to you in the New Year' in big letters on the board on the bottom landing, I winced. When he drove up to my parents' house in Stockport to bring me back to Wakefield after his Boxing Day shift, and sat with his hand firmly on my knee while he chatted to my mum and dad, I accepted his eagerness to return me to his home turf, and this physical display of ownership, as affection. But

I would soon come to recognize it as control. I mistook a number of his early behaviours as romantic, another subliminal consequence, perhaps, of all of the films I'd watched with my gran as child – watching her swoon at John Wayne in *The Quiet Man*, as he wrestles Maureen O'Hara into a wind-swept and violent kiss, even though she is clearly trying her hardest to escape him.

*

In 2006, Prison Officer John Hall was arrested, convicted and sentenced to life imprisonment. Over a period of eight years, while he had been the senior officer at Wakefield, including the time I was working there, he had raped four women, including a work colleague. When one of the women he attacked begged him to stop, he punched her so hard in the face that he dislocated her jaw. He had also kidnapped and sexually assaulted three girls, the youngest of whom was just 12 years old. He'd persuaded them to get in his car and then driven them to deserted places where he locked the doors, forcibly pulled their clothes down, groped them and masturbated himself in front of them. After his arrest, police found child-abuse images on his computer. Hall used his warrant card and usually wore his prison officer's uniform during these attacks, passing himself off as a policeman. I heard through the grapevine that colleagues of Hall's were apparently shocked to their core by his arrest. It brought to mind the phrase toads in hot water. Maybe we had all been toads in hot water at HMP Wakefield during that time. Some were bigger toads than others.

People don't always come with a warning sign. The truth is that the outfit might be different, they might be behind bars, they might be patrolling the streets. They might have families and careers, hold positions of authority and trust. They might be someone you know. But civilized society has such fixed ideas about who criminals are – we carry around our internalized profiles of the law-breakers, existing in negative relief to us, the good ones. And one of the many consequences when we psychologically divorce ourselves from them in this way, dehumanize them even, consider them monsters, is that we become blind to those who are moving among us.

The truth is that no modesty curtain can be conveniently drawn between them and us. There is no them and us, it is just us.

CHAPTER 2
BIG BOYS DON'T CRY

When we cannot find a way of telling our story,
our story tells us.
Stephen Grosz, *The Examined Life*

Some time before his arrival in prison, Patrick Thompson had tried to kill himself with a shotgun but had missed his brain and blew a chunk of the left side of his face off instead. When he walked into the small interview room that morning, still very much alive, I didn't manage to fully disguise my shock at how he looked. His earlobe, some of his jaw and most of his cheek were missing, and what remained was a collection of scars and bumps and hollows. The other side of his face seemed disfigured too, almost melted, and his right eye was cloudy. Thankfully he had come prepared with some of his paintings to show me, which provided a welcome diversion for both of us. We spent some moments looking at them, exchanging polite conversation about his work, while we both mentally settled into the unnatural situation in which we found ourselves. I was here to find out if Thompson had any plans to try to kill himself again.

It was a couple of years after my first research post in Wakefield that I found myself in jail again, this time doing a brief stint as a locum on the healthcare wing of a category B local prison. Most jails have a healthcare wing or unit, where sick or injured prisoners are held and treated by prison nurses and (if they are lucky and can find one) visiting doctors. It is no exaggeration to say that the units, by and large, are warehouses of human suffering. At any time there will be a mix of prisoners who are physically ill, some terminal and dying, others injured through violence or self-harm, those who are dangerously drunk or high, or experiencing severe withdrawal from their addictions. People in the healthcare unit are at their lowest depths, mentally and physically. Even the smell is desperate – a blend of disinfectant, sweat, vomit and every other human discharge imaginable. The sound is haunting, too. In any prison you'll generally notice a continual background drone of chatter, activity and radios, but a healthcare unit is more often a place of ominous silence, punctuated by immediate and absolute cacophony – shouting, banging, alarm bells, doors clanging, screaming. The things you see and hear in a prison healthcare unit can be profoundly unnerving unless you are used to it. By that time, I was used to it.

On my second day, I was walked up to the interview room by an operational support grade (OSG), a member of the ancillary staff responsible for gate procedures and visitor movements, a round man with a beard and a pot belly who in a different life would have made a great Father Christmas. He was clearly relieved to see an outsider, and talked at me all the way through the corridors and up the stairs, cheerily explaining how most of his workmates were off sick with stress, or had been battered by inmates and were incapacitated.

We went past the safe cell, a space you find in most healthcare wings, with a gate rather than a solid door so the occupant can be observed at all times. There are no sharp edges or things to hang yourself from in a safe cell. Out of my peripheral vision I noticed the inmate inside wave casually at me and I nodded back. The OSG told me that this man had been taken to A & E two nights before, because he'd reopened an old self-inflicted wound on his groin and packed it with dirty toilet paper, so that it had become infected. Apparently the escorting officer, who was handcuffed to the inmate throughout the visit to A & E, thought he just fancied a trip out, or some opiates that he didn't have to pay for, so had told the nurse on duty not to give him any painkillers while they washed out the wound and stitched him up. The prisoner jerked so violently with the agony of the stitches that it had pulled the officer's shoulder straight out of its socket, with an audible pop. My gossipy escort was telling me this story as though it was a hilarious anecdote, but his enthusiasm tailed off as he saw my face hardening into a Queen Victoria scowl.

It was an unforgiving British winter, cold to the bone, and I remember wearing my standard prison 'uniform' of black woollen polo neck and trousers to work most days. The healthcare wing was an extension to the main building, a 1980s block with low ceilings and harsh strip lighting, moulded plastic furniture and the kind of lino flooring that goes halfway up the wall. The rooms were all painted in that drab NHS green that is supposed to be calming but instead evokes a strange kind of despondency. In the small room I was allocated, the table was fixed to the wall (so no one could throw it at you) and the large storage heater, hanging from the wall like a piece of hot Lego, was on full blast. Even if Thompson wasn't intending to kill himself, it felt like we might both roast to death in there.

The low staff numbers weren't a surprise. New, tougher sentencing legislation meant prisoner counts were creeping up, but at the same time what would become savage cutbacks to staffing budgets were being introduced, and the pace of new prison building was far shy of demand. The chronic overcrowding, and the squalor that comes with it, that I have come to think of as normal in prisons today, was just starting to take hold at this place. I always say that, unless they have inordinate powers of self-awareness, the workforce ends up taking on the characteristics of the people they are responsible for. The staff here were clearly overwhelmed, feeling unsupported and losing the will to carry on.

With overcrowding and understaffing, nearly all offender-rehabilitation work had ground to a halt. When rehab stops there is no work or education, no therapy groups or counselling. Prisoners have less meaningful contact with staff and each other, spending more time on lockdown in their cells (in theory alone, but there were very few inmates alone in a cell here – more like three crammed in at a time, the world's worst game of sardines). Lockdown contains people, but it can also mentally shut them down. As the Nobel Prize-winning poet Joseph Brodsky put it: 'Prison is essentially a shortage of space made up for by a surplus of time; to an inmate, both are palpable.' For prisoners spending up to 23 hours a day on lockdown there is no purpose, no stimulation and, most brutal: no hope. At this prison, a very real sense of hopelessness – the psychological precursor to suicide – pervaded the air.

Suicide is a big problem in prison. The basic duty of care to keep people alive isn't as simple as it should be. Along with one of the highest prison populations, we also have one of the highest prison suicide rates in Europe. (Suicide was still illegal in the UK until 1961, which is why we still hear talk of people 'committing' suicide. Oddly enough, I've never worked with anyone with a conviction for killing themselves.) In England and Wales, male prisoners are up to six times more likely to die by suicide than their unincarcerated counterparts, and suicide rates in female prisoners are 20 times higher than in women on the outside. It's not a decision that comes easily, to end your life. The majority of prisoners show signs of significant mental disturbance; the Prison Reform Trust estimates 70 per cent. How many come in like that or start to struggle once there is unclear. But even a short sentence – nearly half of all UK prisoners go in for six months or less – makes a person far more likely to develop mental health problems in the future. Like a trip to Ikea, it's almost impossible to leave without something.

So there was a very real sense at this prison that the ship was sinking. The work of what was left of the staff had become about throwing the water out, trying to stay afloat. Prisons follow a procedure to monitor inmates who are considered to be at risk of harming or killing themselves. Certain forms should be continuously updated by a nurse or prison officer, someone who sees the inmate day to day and knows them, but with a skeletal staff and the number of inmates causing concern so high, I'd been brought in to help wade through the sheer volume of open cases. If they hadn't already disappeared, any lofty ideas I had about the rehabilitation of offenders were about to get a reality check.

I was a kind of one-woman pop-up clinic for inmates, operating from a glorified, and very hot, cupboard in the healthcare wing. I was here to ask questions, observe and look for red flags that might predict a suicide attempt: had a relationship on the outside stalled, were they being bullied, how were they feeling, had they made a plan to kill themselves? These questions are standard, and important, but can feel perfunctory, as someone planning to end their life may not want to share these details with a random woman they've just met in an overheated box room. Besides, as if being in prison isn't enough, the triggers conspiring to drive someone over the edge are often too numerous and varied to point at and say: It was this. You can rarely be that certain.

*

Patrick was brought up to see me from his normal location on B wing. I'd had only a brief moment to glance at his form beforehand. It had been created three weeks ago, after he had tried to hang himself with a makeshift noose fashioned from his bed sheet – the preferred method for most suicides in prison.

I sensed he had brought his pictures with him as a way of deflecting attention from his face, and that he was aware of how people instinctively reacted. I was grateful to him for it. Art is a surprisingly common activity inside – something absorbing that everyone can do peacefully in their cells, and which isn't pornographic or illegal. The paintings reminded me of Van Gogh on a bad day; thick, dauby brush strokes, portraits of unknown men and women, the obligatory fruit bowl, landscapes of green fields with trees and familiar-looking coastlines. They were homely, traditional subjects painted in the sort of splodgy, semi-abstract style that comes into better focus the further away you stand. He told me he painted with his left hand, although he was naturally right-handed – he was missing his index, middle and ring finger on that side. I wondered what had happened to them, but I didn't ask. After we'd looked at the pictures I propped them up against the wall behind us and we got on with the assessment interview.

His responses were flat and monosyllabic, almost predictable. He seemed to put all his energy into just getting the answers out, without making much eye contact with me or expanding on anything. He was clearly uncomfortable being asked to reveal anything personal and was shutting me down with the brevity of his replies. When I asked if he was still having thoughts about killing himself, there was only an almost imperceptible quick nod and flare of the nostrils. I was, after all, a perfect stranger to him, and here I was asking him if he wanted to die.

Having gone through all the questions, I concluded that Patrick's mood remained low, his 'at risk' form should remain open and that he should stay in the shared cell he was in on the normal wing. Any change to his present management – increased observation (hello safe cell) or other safety measures – was likely to be demeaning and counter-productive. Realistically, they'd also be practically impossible with the crisis that the prison was in.

Feeling that he wasn't going to say much more and with an eye on the clock – I had 20 of these reviews to plough through – I got up to retrieve his pictures from behind me.

That's when I realized they had melted. I had propped Patrick's paintings up against the raging hot wall heater and now gooey dribbles of paint were sliding down from the canvases onto the lino floor. The plastic pouch they'd been in had also melted, and was stuck to the wall heater like a piece of bad shrink wrap.

My first thought was simply, Fuck! This man's pride and joy had been gently simmered into a custard and it was all my fault. I had arrived this morning on a mission to preserve lives and now I was about to be responsible for triggering even greater despair. I couldn't speak; I was trying to pull the pictures apart slowly, hoping to salvage something from the wreckage, but also aware of a terrible nervous impulse to laugh. I knew he was watching me, and when I looked at him and he saw the mortified look on my face something wonderful happened: he burst out laughing. For a moment I wasn't actually sure it was laughter. It was an unfamiliar, rasping sound – the result of his facial injuries. But then he picked up one of the melted portraits and held it next to his own face, the scurrilous implication being that it looked like him. He was trying to make me feel better.

I couldn't help myself, I erupted too. We were both really giggling now, in that side-clutching way that you just can't stop. Just as the laughter tailed off we both glanced at each other and set off again – in genuine hysterics. I kept apologizing.

A nurse looked in through the observation panel in the door and then popped her head inside, just to make sure everyone was all right. Her shocked-slash-disapproving expression from behind the door made her look for a split second like Kenneth Williams in *Carry On Matron*. It must have been an unusual sound, me and him roaring with laughter – real belly laughs aren't that common in prison, even in the unpredictable healthcare environment. And this was supposed to be a suicide risk assessment.

I learned the value of humour in my work in that moment. Sometimes in the most inappropriate situations it is the only appropriate response. Spend time with any emergency services teams, and you'll hear gallows humour as a means of coping in the bleakest situations. But in psychology and mental health, laughter with a patient or client can still feel somehow wrong, unrestrained, too improper. The popular image of a psychologist is someone buttoned-up and coolly analytical; as forensic trainees we are taught to remain professionally distant. But it can also make you seem like an automaton. Boundaries need to be maintained, of course, but not at the expense of being authentic.

In laughing uncontrollably about this man's melted paintings, I was breaking unwritten rules about letting go in this kind of exchange. But, between you and me, I have always loved a good joke at the wrong moment, if it is done kindly and at no one's expense – as they say, laughing with people not at them. It can be a very effective tool. Laughter is the best tension diffuser I know. There is a place for it even, as it turns out, in a suicide assessment. This moment with Patrick was a real and harmless way to respond in the situation, and its effects turned out to be remarkable.

Patrick started to cry. I quickly reached for the box of tissues I always have on the table for this kind of moment (although no inmate would usually ever have dreamed of using them in front of me). He said he wasn't crying because of the pictures, but because of 'everything else'. I looked at the clock, knowing this would put me behind schedule, but I didn't want to stop him, so I asked him to tell me about it. This overly controlled man, who had been so hard to read a few minutes ago, was opening up, prompted by that little bit of human connection and a shared moment of vulnerability. I wasn't going to stop him now.

Patrick – in his late 50s, not an especially tall man but wide, almost square, with stocky limbs and a chubby neck – had worked as a night-time security guard at an agricultural warehouse in the middle of the countryside where he lived. He'd grown up in this rural region, where the landscape was wide open and life happened quietly in the villages, people connected by lanes and fields. In his job, Patrick spent his nights in a small office attached to the side of the warehouse, guarding the big farming machinery that made the community tick. It wasn't anyone's dream job, but there was certainly purpose in his work.

One night the warehouse owner, Patrick's employer, started a fire at the building in an attempt to cash in on his insurance. He had switched off the fire alarms, so the first Patrick knew about the blaze raging through the place was the smell of smoke as it crept under his office door. He described how he had leaped into action, rushing from his desk to open the door to the main storage, but a violent backdraft lifted him off his feet in a blast of hot ash and flames, and threw him across the room. Patrick had suffered severe injuries: burns to his face and his right arm, and three fingers lost on his right hand. He was, everyone agreed, lucky to have survived.

The warehouse owner spent a short time in prison for his crime and Patrick spent a long time in and out of hospital, having a series of painful plastic surgery operations and skin grafts. Unable to even talk properly because of the surgery to his face, he had literally been muted. Over this drawn-out and difficult period, his wife left him. She moved out of their home while he was in hospital.

A few months after returning home to his new reality, he tried to kill himself with his own shotgun (it was legally held, quite usual in farming communities). He put the gun in his mouth hoping for a clean end, but without an index finger to pull the trigger he had, miraculously, managed not to kill himself. Instead, he had blown off part of his face – mostly the part that hadn't already been damaged in the fire. More painful surgery and weeks of silent agony in hospital followed for him – all the time knowing he had no one to go home to.

Patrick, heavily disfigured, unemployed and alone, decided he was going to have it out with his former employer. He went to the man's house, after a few too many drinks one night, with the intention of settling the score. But it had gone further than that. He'd picked up a log from a woodpile by the front door and hit him repeatedly with it. Then he'd given him a kicking while he was on the ground. He admitted that at one point it had stopped being a person he was hitting, it was just his own pain. Patrick said that, for a brief moment, he had felt better. But then he looked at the near-dead man on the floor and understood what he had done. He used the man's phone to call the ambulance.

This wasn't an impulsive, recklessly angry man, the type that goes around punching everyone he meets. Patrick was the opposite. He was over-controlled, emotionally contained. Anger can be adaptive and healthy, if it is handled well, but he bottled his up and let it grow into a poison tree, until he had erupted into a cathartic rage – cathartic for a short time, anyway. It's usually the case that this type of person commits infrequent acts of violence – maybe even just once in a lifetime – but is more likely to seriously hurt, maybe kill, a victim when they do.

Now Patrick was on remand, awaiting what was undoubtedly going to be a long sentence for causing grievous bodily harm. Hopelessness was alive and well in him.

*

Telling our personal stories, naming and acknowledging our experiences, is fundamentally how human beings make sense of our world. For most of us that means talking with our friends or family. For others it's therapy or counselling – the premise is the same: through the simple act of talking we process and understand ourselves, and others. When we don't or can't tell our stories, they manifest in other ways. Emotions need a voice. Without it they seep out eventually.

But the art of talking comes easier to some of us than others. For boys and men, so many of them still socialized in a myriad of destructive ways to hide weakness and tough out their difficulties, the idea of sharing deep emotional pain with anyone is still often unthinkable, even in the 21st century. When you are punished or mocked if you dare to express, or even have, feelings, you typically put a lot of effort into appearing strong and stoic. Except for anger. Male conditioning is more accepting of anger, an emotion that is usually more about 'doing' than 'feeling'. Men are, generally speaking, more likely to deal with distress by doing something: overworking, sex, drinking, drugs, aggression, violence, suicide. What is suicide if not the most decisive of actions, after all. Small wonder then that the ultra-macho prison environment, where having emotions is seen as a sign of weakness, is full of men acting out their distress in harmful ways.

*

Patrick Thompson didn't know how to tell his story, with all its trauma and tragedy. He just couldn't have found the moment, even if he'd been given the chance to, which he hadn't, not before he'd committed a serious crime, and certainly not after. Listen hard enough and even the quietest prisons are booming with the deafening sound of men not talking.

There was something of my own that I wasn't talking about at that time, keeping under wraps, unacknowledged even to myself. But my unspoken story was beginning to manifest itself in a physical way – I'd started to have attacks of dizziness. One evening at Sheffield railway station I collapsed out of nowhere. People assumed I was drunk. It felt like I was drunk, or had the mother of all hangovers, just without any of the fun or cocktails. I was on the platform, waiting to board a train home to Manchester. Suddenly the train in front of me seemed to move backwards, and before I had time to think about why it would be doing that, the whole platform started to spin and I fell over. I was trying to grip the floor, holding on to it because it felt like a cyclone had struck platform 14. I was momentarily transported back to the waltzer at the Red Rec in Stockport, where we went as teenagers when the fair came to town. I could hear voices around me but couldn't speak because it was taking all my mental effort to breathe through the panic and nausea, trying to grasp a sense of balance. Attacks like this were starting to become more frequent.

I was grateful to Patrick for the laughter that day. I realized I had needed that release of tension just as much as he had. For a moment I worried that I had kicked a man while he was down, and maybe even made him more likely to want to end his life. But as we gathered up the melting plastic pouch and what was left of his art, he thanked me. I asked him if I needed to be more concerned about him. He smiled his one-sided smile and said, 'No, not today. It won't be today.'

He wanted to stay alive that day and, sometimes, in this job, just helping a person hang on until the next moment is good enough. I never saw Patrick again. I hope he found a way to keep on talking, and made it to the end of his sentence.

CHAPTER 3
THE BLAME GAME

The just-world hypothesis: The widespread but false belief that the world is essentially fair, so that the good are rewarded and the bad punished. One consequence of this belief is that people who suffer misfortunes are assumed to deserve their fates…even the victims often blame themselves.
Oxford Dictionary of Psychology

I'll always remember Alison because she is the only person I've seen walk out of Crown Court a free woman after being convicted of killing her husband.

It was 2003 and the first time I'd been asked to act as an expert witness in a homicide case (although it sounds American, 'homicide' is a generic term that when used in the UK covers murder, manslaughter and infanticide). Because we assess people and not the objects pertinent to a case, psychologists are among a small number of professionals who are permitted to give their two penn'orth in court, rather than just report on the facts of a matter. I was 29, and I'd reached a level of experience and professional standing that meant I was now being trusted to provide opinions that had huge ramifications not only for the people on trial, but for the family of the victim and the public.

I had always assumed this milestone case for me would involve a male defendant. No gender stereotyping intended, it's just an indisputable fact that 95 per cent of our killers are male, regardless of relationship, if any, between victim and perpetrator. Men are overwhelmingly killed by other men, and women are also overwhelmingly killed by men. So when the file came through from the Crown Prosecution Service with the request to accept instructions, I was surprised to see I'd been asked to assess a female defendant.

Alison was currently charged with murder, having admitted to killing her husband, Paul, at their home. What the CPS wanted to know was what kind of mental state Alison was in at the time and, specifically, did she have an 'abnormality of mental functioning' on the day she killed him that had 'caused, or significantly contributed to her conduct'. This question, posed in legal-speak, made it clear that Alison's team were putting forward a defence of diminished responsibility, and would be hoping to get her charge reduced to manslaughter.

We are still a civilized society, so the foundation for criminal law is that a person is guilty only if proved to be blameworthy in both their conduct (known as *actus reus*: the guilty act) and their intention, or appreciation of the act being wrong (their ability to form the necessary *mens rea*: guilty mind). An insufficient *mens rea* is the general difference between murder and manslaughter. But to establish what the state of Alison's mind was in the exact moments that she killed Paul, we needed to make a retrospective evaluation, a difficult thing to do with the degree of certainty required in law. Being able to travel back in time is one of the many additional skills a forensic psychologist needs on their CV.

I immediately put in a request for her medical records and booked out several hours of visiting sessions with her at the women's prison where she was being held on remand. While preparing to take my first look at the prosecution evidence and plan my assessment of Alison, I took a moment to reflect on what I knew about 'intimate partner homicide'.

Paul was in the approximately 10 per cent of all victims who are men killed by the women in their life. Just 1 per cent of victims are women killed by other women. Research also tells us over and over that when men kill their female partners or ex-partners, it usually follows months or years of them abusing her. On the other hand, when women kill their husbands or exes, it's usually after months or years of having been abused by the man they have killed.

This is usually the point at which someone pops up, like Cato Fong out of a cupboard in *The Pink Panther*, to attack my apparent misandry and point out that men are also victims of domestic abuse. Of course there are male victims, and every case must be taken seriously. Nevertheless, domestic abuse is a gendered crime in that it disproportionately happens to women and is mostly perpetrated by men. It is women who are more likely to experience the more severe forms of emotional abuse and control, and be subject to repeated and long-term victimization. And women are far more likely to be seriously hurt, or worse, by someone who once professed to love them. Violent men put a woman in hospital in Britain every three hours. These are the ugly but irrefutable facts.

I knew there was a strong probability that Alison had been abused by Paul, possibly over a long period of time. However, I can't make an assessment or form any kind of opinion based on probabilities. So I set aside statistics as I opened the first of three blue folders of crime scene evidence and began to immerse myself in Alison and Paul's case.

*

Looking at crime scene pictures is always a strange thing, intruding on something so personal as someone's death, albeit through the lens of your professional curiosity. They are usually images of intense dissonance: you have the common, everyday banality of the setting – in this case Paul and Alison's red-brick semi, with shrubs in the driveway and stained glass in the uPVC front door – contrasted with the horror of the crime that has taken place there. For Paul it turned out that meant being killed by blunt-force trauma to the head and then stabbed in the chest while he lay on the sofa.

My first thoughts, as I looked through these pictures, were that I wasn't seeing anything like an organized or premeditated crime scene. It was a vision of chaos. In the living room, where he had been killed, Paul's body lay on the floor, his bare lower legs and feet sticking out from the duvet – or was it two duvets? – he had been messily bundled up in. In the background stood a Christmas tree, a festive symbol of evergreen life and familial bliss, covered in swathes of silver tinsel, behind it shelves with picture frames and the odd figurine.

The pictures took me on a tour of the events that had unfolded. His face and a large part of his head were caked in blood and the left eye was heavily swollen, a plum-coloured contrast to the rest of his skin. There was an unmistakable expression of shock on his face. He had obviously had a split second to register what was about to happen to him. His hand, locked into a claw shape, was by his face, as though it had shot up in that moment to protect himself. I took in the stab wounds on his chest but they were small, colourless slits, like fingernail marks in the skin of an apple. There was no blood, they were just entry wounds, indicating they'd happened after he had died. Pictures of his torso showed where she'd apparently tried, not very effectively, to cut him in half at the waist – again no sign of bleeding just the carved flesh, standing proud. There were bin bags and cleaning sponges in some pictures and a toilet roll on the carpet. In the kitchen, what looked like human excrement. A washing-up bowl in the sink with a wrench in it, the water reddish brown.

This wasn't so much a cover-up job as a clean-up job – a futile one at that. I've seen plenty of homicide scenes over the years and I've learned that the body of someone who has met a premature death is a difficult, laborious thing to clean up after, even for the most methodical, scientific of killers. The person who had sponged the sofa and tried to lift the blood splatters off the carpet with toilet roll clearly didn't have the kind of strength or calculated thinking required to disguise their actions. Having made an abortive attempt to move and cut into Paul's body, Alison had wrapped him up in duvets, no longer able to bear looking at what she had done. And there he remained on the light floral carpet.

Other pictures in the house showed an entirely average, if unusually neat and clean, home. The children's bedrooms bore none of the mess and chaos of most kids' rooms. Dolls were lined up in uniform rows on shelves, more for display than playing with. In the main bedroom an ironing board was up and shirts hung up on wardrobe doors. The bed, with full pelmet and more dolls, was immaculately made. I was struck by the perfection of the front drive – no leaves, no plant pots or any of the usual disarray of family life, like someone had vacuumed the asphalt. Next to the house was a garage full of all the usual garage miscellanies: tools and paint, a workbench. Underneath a shelf of household products, bleach and disinfectants, was a shelf full of alcohol – five or six big bottles of vodka and other spirits.

And then the note. She'd torn pages from a child's flowered notebook, and written on both sides, although not in the lines. The writing looked sketchy, with thin spidery letters, written by a hand that was obviously shaking. It said: 'It can't go on like this, I can't cope any more. I'm sorry. Please look after the children, tell them I love them. They are with my mum, please let them stay with my mum.' It said the same thing over all four pages: sorry and I couldn't cope any more. There was no linear thought process or considered structure here. It was a stream of consciousness that had burst out of her, there and then. She lay down next to Paul's body on the floor and stayed there until her mum came round the next morning with the children.

The prison she was being held in was the same, in essence, as the other women's prisons I'd been to. There are only 12 dedicated women's prisons in England (women make up just 10 per cent of the UK prison population). They are absolutely nothing like the sassy world portrayed in American TV shows like *Orange Is the New Black*. For one thing there are no boiler suits and women wear their own clothes in British jails – if there is a uniform it's denim and T-shirts, comfort over style. The rooms where I've spent time with female prisoners are largely similar to those in men's prisons, but there are also sometimes more pleasant rooms in women's prisons, with bright pictures on the walls and boxes of toys, like a dentist's waiting room. Only those rooms are where mothers wait to see their children.

I met Alison in this kind of family room. It had a little kitchenette area with a sink and a cluster of low, padded chairs. I remember the lights were on a movement sensor, and because we were sat so low down I had to flap my arms around every 15 minutes to stop them going out, an irritating necessity that felt inappropriately slapstick given the gravity of what I was here to discuss with her.

She was thin, average height, her hair was scraped back in a harsh ponytail, with slender features and wide-set brown eyes. I noticed flecks of grey and thinned-out patches around her temples, and little dents on her ears where the earrings had long-since been taken out. As she talked her eyes were glossy with tears, which fell slowly and steadily throughout our conversation.

She told me that the first time Paul had hurt her was when she told him she was pregnant, ten years ago. They were sitting in their car, him in the passenger seat, and he smashed her face into the steering wheel. It had happened so quickly that at first she thought that another car had hit them from behind. When she told her mother, she asked what Alison had done to provoke him and told her that, if she was pregnant, she had made her bed and had better lie in it. She later lost the baby when Paul pushed her down the stairs, although he told her it was her imagination, she would have lost the baby anyway. This is a tactic known as 'gaslighting' – when an abuser manipulates their victim into doubting their own perceptions and sanity.

She had called the police on three occasions, but no action was taken nor had charges been brought. She said that after the third time Paul gave her such a beating in punishment she didn't dare report him again. Join any discussion on domestic abuse, and you'll hear someone ask why women don't just leave or call the police. It sounds so simple. But the dynamic between two people in an abusive relationship is incredibly intense, a spinning wheel of violence and shock, deep remorse, emotionally powerful reconciliations, hope and elation. And then the terror. After a period of calm the victim knows something is coming, they just don't know when, and they attempt to see it off by changing their behaviour – going 'into' themselves, disappearing, doing whatever it takes to keep the peace. But they never can. And inevitably there is more violence, and the cycle begins again.

For both parties in this potent loop, each repetition of the cycle propels them to the next. The victim adapts quickly, as the threat of violence creates a strong incentive to learn. She begins to believe that her circumstances are a result of her personal failure, and views herself as worthless, weak. When she is a good girl, it will stop. Until then, she doesn't deserve anyone else's love. The abuser also becomes attached to the power they hold, and the skilful use of violence and manipulation to achieve the deference that they expect from their partner. This wretched dynamic is like a scar tissue that meshes them together. So leaving, while it may appear like an obvious course of action to many, often feels impossible for the victim.

Alison had found a much sought-after place at a women's refuge, but Paul had followed her and forced her to come home, threatening to tell social services just how mad she was and that they'd take away her children. Alison had a habit of cleaning, meticulously and repeatedly cleaning. He said that she'd get locked up if people knew about it.

She explained that she'd worked in a restaurant as a teenager, and the place had been temporarily closed down because it had breached food hygiene regulations. Her mother – an exacting woman who she could never please – had suggested that she couldn't have possibly been doing her job properly, and the compulsion to clean crept in. Rituals that had later grown into something she did when she was feeling anxious, a way of trying to impose order on the chaotic stream of worry in her mind, which by this stage in her life occupied every waking moment. She described how Paul would torment her by crushing packets of biscuits and crisps and scattering the contents around the house.

Her medical records showed she had been admitted to hospital more than a few times over the past couple of years with unexplained injuries – once for burns to her throat after drinking bleach. At the time she'd told doctors it was an accident. When I asked her about it she told me that Paul had forced her to drink it one day when he'd become irritated by her cleaning. He'd forced his hand over her mouth and held her nose to make her swallow it. The doctors knew that this was no accident – I've certainly never met an adult who drinks bleach by mistake – and they asked her if she needed to tell them anything. But she had stayed quiet, too scared of her children being taken away if she said anything. A nurse came to talk to her but, getting nowhere, ended the conversation by implying that if Alison kept 'going back to that, she must enjoy it'.

Alison told me he raped her. She said that on Saturday afternoons he would get obliterated with the vodka from the garage and then would usually expect to have sex. If Alison didn't seem enthusiastic he would force himself on her anyway. If she didn't look like she was enjoying herself, he would sometimes strangle her until her vision blurred and she felt light-headed.

*

On the night she killed him, Alison said she hadn't slept properly for days – things had been calm for a while but the tension was building – she couldn't stop memories of previous assaults from rushing to the front of her mind and sucking the breath from her throat. She said she felt jumpy that afternoon, on eggshells, but also worn out with the effort of trying not to antagonize him and of trying to stop herself cleaning. She had cried a little bit and he told her to stop ruining his mood. She went into the kitchen so he couldn't see her, and he shouted to her from where he was lying on the sofa, 'Bring me a bottle from the garage.'

This was when she had lost control of her bowels – I had noted the evidence of this in the pictures from the kitchen. In her soiled trousers, shaking with fear, she walked to the garage and, standing in front of the bottles of vodka, she had reached down and picked up a pipe wrench instead. She described how at that moment her terror turned her 'numb, like I was floating'. She turned around and walked straight into the lounge, and standing just behind Paul, who was prone on the sofa with his eyes closed, brought the wrench down onto his head with all the strength she could muster. She couldn't remember precisely how many times she had done it.

She drew in breath as she told me this, visibly horrified by what she had just said. Then she said: 'Poor Paul, poor Paul.'

He was motionless. She could hardly explain it, but said it still seemed to her like he was jumping up at her in a rage, yet he wasn't actually moving. She could only recall jumbled thoughts and panic; she had run back into the kitchen and grabbed a small serrated knife from the knife block and stood there, holding it in front of her for what seemed like a long time, expecting him to burst through at any moment. When she went tentatively back into the lounge she shook him to see if he was alive. Even though it was only because she had shaken him, the movement of his body had terrified her and she punched down on his chest, stabbing him. But he was dead already by then.

Looking down at her hands, she began to say 'Poor Paul' again, but before the words could come she threw up.

*

Sitting in the traffic on the long drive home, nudging slowly along the familiar grey vistas of the motorway, I thought about how I recognized the classic cycle of abuse she described to me. I recognized it not only from the many hours I'd spent studying the dynamics of domestically abusive relationships, but from my own experience.

After I'd left HMP Wakefield I'd continued to see the prison officer. But it had quite quickly turned sour. His behaviour became increasingly domineering and frightening, when I didn't dress as he wanted, fill the kettle from the right tap, put a smile on my face like he wanted or go along enthusiastically with sex as and when *he* wanted. It was what we now refer to as coercive control, I can spot it at 30 paces these days. But hindsight is a wonderful thing, and back then we didn't have a word for it. The onset was so insidious that I may not have identified it, even if we had.

It became intolerable when I started my new job as a trainee forensic psychologist in a hospital secure unit. This kind of opportunity didn't come up very often in those days and I was proud of myself for landing it; I'd made the transition from student volunteer to fully paid, fledgling psychologist. Our relationship had started to feel like the fly in the ointment of my life. I desperately wanted out, but also knew that the moment when an abusive relationship ends is when the risk of harm increases.

I eventually managed to leave, but he didn't want to make it easy for me to go. He began to turn up at my work. Colleagues would tell me he was lingering in the car park or had marched into the reception area demanding to know if I had left the building for the day. He'd bang on the front door or his face would appear at the window of my home at the same time as the phone would start ringing off its hook. I closed the curtains, and sat immobilized until he eventually went away.

On a typically dismal 31 October – Halloween – I'd arrived home from work in the evening and run in to the house just as it was starting to rain. I saw trick or treaters down the road and in a mean-spirited moment thought to myself that they'd be getting soaked in a minute. I rushed in through the door, threw my coat down in the hall and went straight into the kitchen to see if my housemate was home – she wasn't. When the doorbell rang, I practically skipped to the door, expecting to see the painted faces and plastic masks of children. It wasn't them.

*

A few days later it was my housemate who made me call the police, with the ultimatum that if I didn't, she would. It is bloody difficult to make that phone call. I was filled with foreboding about setting in motion the chain of events I knew would follow.

Because when a victim of domestic abuse makes that decision, and calls the police, they are starting a story with only two possible endings, neither of them happy: either the authorities decide not to take action, and hell waits for its dues at home; or action *will* be taken, and they will have to face a new reality – their life and everything they know, upended and dispersed. All I really wanted was for him – everything – to go away. Reporting a crime felt like inviting a whole new wave of problems into my life. Still, I called them, and many months later found myself in court.

Dr Albert von Schrenck-Notzing was the first psychologist known to have testified in court when he gave evidence about the credibility of witness testimony in a Munich murder trial in 1896. I'd been imagining my first moment in court since what seemed like 1896. In my vision I was the erudite expert, holding the court in thrall as I educated judge and jury with my accomplished testimony, Queen's Counsel sighing 'no further questions Your Honour', conceding defeat in the face of my professionalism under cross-examination. What I hadn't ever aspired to was giving evidence as the victim, cheeks burning, struggling to phrase my justifications for not complaining sooner.

In the court proceedings that eventually followed, I testified that I felt like a performing seal, constantly trying to keep the mood upbeat and see off a potential rage that could be triggered by something minuscule and, once ignited, could blaze for days. So I understood the state of perpetual fear that Alison talked about – always expectant, waiting for something to blow up and doing everything you can to avoid it – but finding over and over again that you can't, because of course it isn't your behaviour that is the problem, it is theirs.

It was only a local magistrates' court – small, so no jury, just three magistrates, me, my ex-boyfriend and his legal advocate, a prosecutor, but also what appeared to be an assembly of the entire nation's press. His solicitor

– doing his job – asked me a series of personal and embarrassing questions about the relationship we'd had. This was a man I had had an on-and-off relationship with, had been intimate with, after all. Wasn't I making a big fuss about nothing? Surely this was a lovers' tiff? The over-reaction of an attention-seeking, hysterical young woman. I was a timewaster, a liar – at least that was what I was being told.

He was convicted of harassment two weeks later, and sentenced to 18 weeks in prison, of which he could expect to serve nine. In actual fact, he only spent a weekend in prison; after the trial his solicitor sprang into action, arguing that as a prison officer he was in too much danger from other inmates – and his sentence was later dropped on appeal.

Media reporting of crime and actual events so often seem to exist in different dimensions, entirely unconnected by truth or facts. Newspapers sell stories and stories get spun to suit their agenda. This episode had all the salacious elements of the perfect tabloid story – the prison officer and the redhead. Of course that was how this tale was going to play out in the tabloids.

When I caught that surreal first glimpse of myself on a news-stand as I went to work that morning I felt suddenly unsteady, like I was in a lift that was going down too fast. When I walked into the communal ward area, where all the papers were laid out on the table every day, there I was on the front page of most of the tabloids. One had gone with a classic prison pun about the warden who got his *lag over* with the firecracker shrink. Another had dedicated two full pages to the story. Referring to a very difficult piece of evidence I'd given, they'd opted for a lurid description of his scrawling across my naked breasts in lipstick – he'd actually written 'feminist bitch' on me. I was stunned at the time that a man would turn me into a human graffiti wall (and that he knew how to spell feminist) and I remain stunned to this day that this most personal detail of my testimony was repurposed by a journalist as cheap titillation.

It is very difficult to describe shame. I'd been gradually getting a measure of how deep it cuts via my clients – both the victims and the ones who had done terrible things to others. But perhaps it is something you have to feel in order to fully appreciate it. I went to the toilets and stood looking at myself in the mirror, sick at my own image.

My supervisor could see I was in no state to work and told me to go home. Almost as an afterthought he said: 'But before you do, you need to go and apologize to Dr Wilcox.' Dr Wilcox was the consultant psychiatrist whose team I was attached to. I should go and show my remorse to my superiors, like a kid who had stolen a biscuit. They weren't angry, just disappointed. Unquestioning, I barrelled into his office and babbled a nonsensical apology. The man clearly didn't know what on earth was going on and got me out of there as quickly as he could. I'll never forgive my supervisor for further humiliating me that day. He was a generally decent and supportive man who I otherwise enjoyed working with, but on that particular occasion sensitivity deserted him.

When I came back to work a day or two later, no one in the staff room mentioned it. Not one colleague. Everyone knew about it by that stage but no one said a word, it was eyes down in every office I walked into. My colleagues – highly skilled nurses and psychologists – didn't see past the headlines. Or if they did they never told me, or asked how I was feeling. Their discomfort was palpable. The subtext was that this wasn't how we did things, we were mental health professionals and this was something that happened to our patients, not us. All I could do was try to keep my head up, but it was hard.

On my first day back I sat down for five minutes alone in the patients' communal area – where the newspapers had been – and three of the female patients approached me. They were holding a small bunch of white daisies, obviously picked from the lawn outside. These women – people with learning difficulties, who heard things, had visions and held unusual beliefs, who were supposedly far out of touch with reality – stood there and handed me these daisies. They didn't say a word but I knew what they were for. They nodded silently at me, and

I nodded back. This little trio had more compassion in that moment than any of the staff – the experts who couldn't even speak to me or look at me.

I was on a yearly renewable contract and, a couple of months later, when my contract wasn't renewed, I knew immediately why. I had been with the hospital for almost two years and there had never been any issue with my work. My ward manager even wrote to the directorial board to express his dismay at my leaving. But the contract wasn't renewed and no explanation was given – none was needed, I wasn't being sacked, after all. There was simply no further requirement for my post. My supervisor told me, off the record, that I had embarrassed the hospital and there was concern about how I had apparently let this happen. They felt I was an inappropriate person to work with some of the male patients who had sexual offence histories (although it was OK for them to share a ward with female patients).

And so I went. I thought that was it; I had messed it all up. I had ended my own career before it had begun. He had returned to his job (a spotless criminal record is on the desirable list on the person specification for prison warden, but isn't actually necessary for the job) but I had somehow lost mine. Not only that, I had humiliated myself in the most public way.

A well-meaning friend gave me her kitten, Serendipity, aka Dippy, to look after for the weekend while she was away. Everyone knows that when you are sad, you need a kitten. Dippy was cute, but as it turned out also part Tasmanian devil, and she spent the weekend ripping every piece of furniture I owned to shreds. Every pot plant got turned upside down and the soil sprinkled liberally across my living-room carpet. When I tried to vacuum up the mess, I realized my Hoover was broken. It was just a bit of soil, but in that moment it was also the last straw. I sat on the floor and sobbed quietly into Dippy's soft fur. My life was a shambles and I couldn't tidy it up.

Oh yes, I appreciated Alison's position. But I wasn't there to empathize. Emotional empathy – not just understanding but *feeling* what another feels – is a beautiful, but also capricious and short-sighted sentiment, not helpful in the professional analysis of the forensic psychologist. It can muddle your thinking and has no place in the context of a forensic evaluation for a court. It is not my job to identify with anyone, no matter how much I might recognize my own story in theirs. None of my experiences and subsequent prejudices are relevant when I am assessing a client.

*

Alison's solicitor sent me copies of the statements taken by police from the couple's neighbours and people who knew them. She was regularly seen with bruises and injuries; in fact, it was common knowledge that Paul hit her. Almost every statement I read said the same thing: I told her to get away, I said she should leave him. No one mentioned telling him to go away, to stop beating her up.

How naturally we seek out and find culpability in the victim. Alison had been told that she was the one at fault long before she had picked up a weapon and become the aggressor.

There was no doubt that Alison was what most people might call a battered wife; hers was a classic case of 'battered wife syndrome'. This depressing term acknowledges the deep and lasting psychological effects of the kind of ongoing, cumulative abuse Alison had endured at Paul's hands. But it's not my preferred terminology; something about it makes it sound almost like a lifestyle choice, like 'stay-at-home mum' with violence. More relevant, it is neither a category of legal defence, nor a recognized diagnostic label in psychiatry.

In the UK we skip between two diagnostic systems: the *Diagnostic and Statistical Manual* (DSM), which is produced by the American Psychiatric Association, and the *International Classification of Diseases* (ICD), produced by the World Health Organization and used throughout Europe. (Even in psychiatry we can't decide who our most special relationship is with.) Battered wife syndrome doesn't appear in either.

So while Alison was clearly a battered woman, I knew this description wouldn't be considered valid in court. Under British law there are a limited number of defences available to someone who stands accused of murder with hopes of having that charge reduced to manslaughter. A 'sudden and temporary loss of control' (what used to be termed 'provocation') is the most commonly used. It's a controversial defence that doesn't tend to offer much hope for abused women.

These days courts accept that ongoing abuse *is* provocation and that its effects might cause someone to react instantly and with violence to what may seem to others like an innocuous trigger. But herein lies the issue: having that instant violent reaction, without simultaneously putting yourself in even greater danger, requires you to be at least as strong as, and ideally more physically dominant than the person provoking you. Not something many abused women can claim to be. An abused woman rarely has the option of a 'sudden and temporary loss of control' while she is being assaulted or threatened, as abusive men are generally bigger and stronger and more terrifying than the women they pick on. An abused woman knows that losing her cool in the heat of the moment may well get her killed.

In effect, the law deems anger, and heated physical actions made in the moment – overwhelmingly the privilege of men in these situations – a real-life get-out-of-jail-free card. It favours those who have their own strength, in immediate supply, to rely on. But, as you might expect, the majority of cases involving women who have killed their abusers feature the use of weapons, most commonly knives, poison or fire.

The case of Sara Thornton brought this issue into the spotlight in 1989. Thornton, from Warwickshire, received a life sentence for the murder of her violent husband after he threatened that she and her ten-year-old daughter would soon be 'dead meat'. The prosecution successfully argued that, because she had taken an estimated 60 seconds to walk into the kitchen and pick up a knife before returning to stab him, her behaviour was premeditated. It was, therefore, outside the 'sudden and temporary' requirement of the loss of control defence. The judge who passed sentence advised that, if she feared for her life, she could have gone outside or upstairs instead. Thornton became the reluctant poster girl for women's justice groups, who felt her case illustrated a deep-set gender bias in the defence options surrounding domestic homicide. That loss of control was a defence for men, written by men, used by men.

Thornton was eventually allowed to appeal and in 1996 had her conviction reduced to manslaughter, with her prison sentence suspended in lieu of the time she'd already served. A victory, of sorts. But Thornton's legal team had argued the appeal by saying that she had a 'personality disorder', and claimed the defence of diminished responsibility. In short, she 'won' her case for leniency only by acknowledging that she was 'sick'.

It was clear to me that Alison had been in an altered state at the time she had killed Paul. Her distress had been building for months. But triggered by his all-too-familiar demand to fetch him a drink, her innate fight-or-flight instincts had kicked in. Powered by the limbic system, the part of the brain that controls our most primitive drives, she turned this time to fight. Her brain sounded an alarm, flooding her with adrenaline and other hormones, sending her sympathetic nervous system into overdrive, mobilizing her body into defensive action.

I wrote a detailed report for Alison, including a 'psychological formulation'. This is a summary for the court of the events of her life, their meaning and relationship to each other. For Alison this was a journey from her childhood, when her mother's criticism had embedded a deep sense of her own low self-worth and guilt, eventually making her easy prey for a controlling man who – over many years – repeatedly beat, raped and humiliated her. On the cusp of yet another assault, her fear was so intense that, for the first time, she fought back.

But to the court a psychological formulation is too broad in its reach. I am required to give my opinion in the specific and accepted language of psychiatry. I wrote that, in my opinion, it was more likely than not that Alison *did* have an abnormality of mind at the time she killed Paul. Specifically, that she reported symptoms that met the criteria for at least three diagnostic labels: 'post-traumatic stress disorder', 'obsessive compulsive disorder' and 'depression'. Although I felt then, and still do, that reducing individual stories to diagnostic 'disorders' like this is like trying to capture the *Mona Lisa* smile with only a painting-by-numbers set at my disposal.

I didn't attend the proceedings in court, but a few weeks later the story came up while I was at home, watching the evening news. There was Alison looking utterly shell-shocked walking out of court, being practically held up by someone who I assumed was her father. The reporter standing outside the Crown Court said Alison had been found guilty of manslaughter on the grounds of diminished responsibility. The court had heard that she had 'killed her husband *because* she was suffering from three different mental illnesses'. The judge had suspended a custodial sentence on condition that she received psychiatric treatment.

I was genuinely surprised Alison hadn't been sent to prison, bearing in mind she had ended a man's life. She shouldn't have killed Paul, but she shouldn't have had to live that way, either. I was satisfied that she would at least get the right help now.

But switching off the television that evening I couldn't shift a niggling feeling of unease. Did Alison really have an abnormality of mind? How abnormal is it to react the way she did? Extreme, undoubtedly. But is it abnormal to react in an extreme way to extreme circumstances? Under different circumstances, if the outcome wasn't so deadly, wouldn't her body's reaction to such a well-established threat be viewed as a normal, useful survival response?

I told myself that it was just a matter of semantics, and tried to put aside the thought that I had been complicit in medicalizing Alison's trauma. As I got into bed and dimmed my bedroom light, I remembered how Paul made Alison believe that the authorities would take her away if they ever found out just how mad she was. The truth was that her reality – the life she lived and all the layers of adversity that she had suffered that ultimately led to her attack on Paul – had been effectively written out of her story. We had conspired to tell the world she had not one, but three mental illnesses. Wasn't this another form of victim blaming?

It was a mental snag that never quite left me, but that I wasn't yet willing to confront.

CHAPTER 4
FAKING IT

All living things contain a measure of madness that moves
them in strange, sometimes inexplicable ways.
Yann Martel, *The Life of Pi*

I held my palms open and showed Travis the 50 pence coin that was sitting in my right hand for a couple of seconds, then clenched my hands shut. I asked him to close his eyes, count backwards from ten and then, 'open your eyes and point to the hand you remember the coin to be in'.

He closed his eyes, his forehead wrinkling in concentration. 'Ten, nine, five, seven.'

I helped him. 'Six, five, four…'

Travis opened his eyes and brought his forefinger up to touch my left hand, then shook his head as I revealed it to be empty. We did this ten times, five with the coin in my right hand and five in the left. He answered wrongly on eight of them.

Inside my mind I allowed myself a little smirk: I knew I was fooling him, even though he thought he was fooling me. I consciously relaxed the muscles in my face, maintaining what I hoped was a concerned and open expression. But I swore I saw a shutter-speed glimpse of a smile – a 'micro-expression' – flash across Travis's face. And then it was gone. There we were, both experiencing our own dose of 'duping delight': the intrinsic pleasure derived from hoodwinking another person, often manifested by the briefest involuntary grin.

This was the coin-in-the-hand test, a so-called 'bedside test', meaning it doesn't need any special equipment or preplanning. It's a short and simple screening exercise designed to help you establish whether a person is feigning memory problems. Very few people can perform badly at this test. It's ridiculously simple. But because it's presented by you – the psychologist – as a difficult task, someone who is faking it will almost always take the opportunity to perform badly, to prove their poor recollection.

Travis had already obtained an exceptionally low score on his IQ test – a standard assessment I do with most of my clients – and yet he was also regularly trouncing members of staff at backgammon, a game which requires considerably more mental agility than his test scores suggested he was capable of. My interest in this curious person was roused and I made a note to keep my eye on him.

I had come across Travis in a medium-secure hospital a few weeks before. He had arrived fresh from prison, in an adapted Leyland DAF van, handcuffed to one of his two escorts. He had been apprehended, several weeks earlier, importing and exporting cheap electronics, a gig which was suspected to be cover for a considerably more lucrative drugs racket. The details were hazy, as Travis claimed to have little recollection of the days leading up to his arrest, or of any of the time he had spent remanded in custody awaiting a trial date.

He was delivered to us under Section 48 of the Mental Health Act, which provides the legal framework for someone to be moved from prison to hospital if their mental health deteriorates to the point that they require a level of care that can't be provided in prison. Travis would have been assessed by two doctors, who would both have been persuaded that he was in such a dire state of mental anguish that he could not remain in prison in the interest of his own wellbeing and safety.

In 1999, this was no mean feat. The information Travis had arrived with was scant but he must have been causing some major concerns at the prison in terms of his behaviour and its management. It is never easy to get a transfer out of prison, except to another prison. Even today, as political interest in mental health issues has grown and a more complex system of funding and service provision makes it mildly more achievable to have severe mental distress recognized, the strategy and protocols set up for the movement of mentally unwell prisoners to secure hospitals are cumbersome and run into long delays. Travis had managed to jump to the front of a queue that others can fester in indefinitely.

This was a relatively new-build extension to an existing hospital and, as is often the case, it was located in the most remote part of the site, away from public gaze. It was a series of low, flat-roofed buildings in bright municipal brick, with decorative external metalwork painted in cheerful primary colours, and small patches of lawn and trees. It could have passed for a leisure centre – one with rather limited facilities – were it not for the six-metre mesh perimeter fence surrounding it.

Like any secure psychiatric facility – places also referred to as forensic hospitals or locked rehabilitation units – many of the people held here had been charged with or convicted of a crime and were deemed too mentally unwell to be in prison. But there were also those who hadn't come into contact with the criminal justice system but whose behaviour was nevertheless considered problematic and too risky for mainstream mental health services.

There were three thirteen-bed wards here and a six-bed long-stay unit for older men, each ward named after an English poet. Most of the men living on Chaucer ward, where I spent most of my working day, were experiencing some form of psychosis: they heard voices or saw things the rest of us didn't. The cast of characters wouldn't have seemed out of place in a Chaucer poem. One man was convinced that I could hear his thoughts and regularly apologized to me for whatever indecorous idea he believed I'd heard pass through his mind. Another patient was adamant that he was here on business; he wore a smart suit every day and kept his room key on a lanyard round his neck. He looked exceptionally convincing, better turned out than any of the real employees, and would welcome visitors to the ward with a firm handshake, introducing himself as the hospital director. Like a plot straight out of a sitcom, several times an unsuspecting hopeful showed up for a job interview that he had somehow managed to arrange while out on his walks in the town, even while being escorted by two members of staff. A third man, a Croatian refugee, believed he was being held by paramilitary forces and was certain that if he could only prove to us his political neutrality he'd be allowed to go home.

Travis didn't exhibit any of these peculiarities, not at first. He settled in quickly and made himself quietly at home. He clearly preferred to make conversation with the female nurses and staff members, in a different setting I may even have described him as a ladies' man. He was immaculately groomed, with a well-trimmed beard, and always smelt fresh, like he'd just spritzed himself with cologne. It was a blazing hot June, and I often saw him sunbathing outside, tapping his foot in beat to the music on his personal stereo, looking for all the world like a student whose exams had just finished.

*

I'd come to work here after finding myself teetering on the verge of unemployment. After hitting the headlines for all the wrong reasons and having my contract at the secure hospital where I'd been working as a trainee 'discontinued', I found myself with less than a month's pay in the bank and only a few weeks left before being out on my ear. I was staring at an uncertain future and wasn't sure what to do with my options, which seemed fairly limited, given that I wasn't yet qualified. Despairing at the prospect of having to return home a failure, and determined not to let my career slip through my fingers, I'd borrowed a copy of the *Forensic Directory* from work and hit the phone, channelling my inner power poser as I began to make calls.

It was a trick I'd learned as a youngster. I was part of the St Winifred's School Choir, which in 1980 somehow managed to have a Christmas number one with a song called 'There's No-one Quite Like Grandma'. It even kept seasonal favourite 'Stop the Cavalry' by Jona Lewie from reaching the top spot. At the height of our popularity, we made a Christmas special for TV, with another 1980s group, The Nolan Sisters. There's a video of it on YouTube, all of us singing 'Have Yourself a Merry Little Christmas' while it snows synthetic snow.

It was the longest day of my then eight-year-old existence and you can see we're all bored, yawning, swaying out of tempo. Somewhere at the front I'm there, slouched over, hands clenched, like a garden gnome that has lost its fishing rod. Just when we thought this interminable day was finally coming to an end, they told us we still had to record a separate soundtrack. Few of us could even speak coherently by that stage, let alone sing, we were out of tune and out of time, more like a funeral than Christmas.

But our headmistress, Sister Aquinas, saved the day. She said: 'Choir, we might not be filming, but you must sing like you are giving the performance of your life. Stand up straight, hold your heads up, put your shoulders back and smile! All the way through this song you must smile!' We all smiled our little faces off and we straight away got the perfect recording.

We had mastered a variant of what Harvard University social psychologist Amy Cuddy would later define as 'power posing'. In her now-famous 2012 TED Talk, she described the art of improving performance via the subtle shifts in brain chemistry and physiology when your mind registers and responds to your body language. The technique has been dismissed as pseudoscience by many, but whether it's a genuine biological lifehack or just the placebo effect, the idea of striking a pose – creating confidence simply by physically affecting it – retains a certain currency. In show business circles they call it 'tits and teeth' (although Sister Aquinas did not call it that) but it all comes down to the same general idea:

fake it until you make it. Whether she knew it or not, Sister Aquinas taught me a valuable life lesson that day.

With the *Forensic Directory* in front of me I started calling the psychiatric hospitals and secure units, beginning with A. Before I'd got even halfway through the alphabet, I had an interview in the diary. I'd asked the hospital manager at this particular medium-secure unit if they had any forensic psychologists on their therapy staff. He said no. I suggested, chancing my arm, that they should have one. He asked me if I was a forensic psychologist and I mumbled something about almost – he told me to hold the line, I heard a muffled exchange, and the following week I was jumping off a train, preparing to grab hold of what looked like the lifeline I needed.

A few weeks and a couple of interviews later, I had a new job – completing my training as a forensic psychologist, and with a pay rise to boot. The hospital manager gave me an old desk and an even older computer, which I could use to finish my master's degree at home in the evenings. I will be forever grateful for that computer, a Macintosh Performa 6200, I'd never have written up my thesis without it. He even had it delivered to my house. I'd rented the nearest place I could find to the hospital, a small, pebble-dashed bungalow with an avocado bathroom suite and an overgrown garden. I had little in the way of possessions back then and the whole place was sparse. But I lived for work, my mind had no space for fripperies or furniture, although I had acquired a cat, a white and tabby rescue given to me by one of the nurses. In the day I would be responsible for setting up the new psychology services, working with my new supervisor, a clinical psychologist who I soon realized was even more keen than I was to build this shiny new department. Even though I said so myself, I had turned things around in spectacular fashion. Sister Aquinas would have been proud.

*

It was my job to carry out the standard assessments on all new patients like Travis, including the IQ assessment, which ideally everyone who was able cooperated with, so that we could rule out any underlying learning disability. I used the Wechsler Adult Intelligence Scale, the gold-standard measure that's been used around the world since it was first created in 1955. It's an essential, and extremely cumbersome, piece of kit comprising a briefcase full of forms, a stopwatch and various props. Intelligence has been defined in many different ways, but Wechsler interprets it as a person's capacity to 'act purposefully, to think rationally, and to deal effectively with his/her environment'. Attempting to capture that, sitting at a table, you ask your client a mixture of questions designed to assess knowledge and memory. There are also some practical performance tests, using pictures, jigsaws and coloured blocks, which help the tester understand a person's capacity for abstract problem-solving.

Throughout the test Travis scratched his head and pursed his lips while drawing in breath sharply, like a contestant on a game show whose answer might win him a million pounds. He assured me that he wanted to do his level best, while also doing all he could to let me know this was an ordeal for him. At the end he had a score of 57; given that the average score of your man-in-the-street is 100, this put him in the extremely low range and flagged up the possibility of a marked learning disability. But a low IQ score can be an indicator of many things.

The way that the Wechsler test is organized means it becomes progressively more demanding until a person's ability to answer correctly reaches a threshold. Typically, right answers tail or drop off abruptly as the tasks get harder. But Travis's answers were patchy and inconsistent. He got some of the easy questions wrong but – just when I thought we could move on to the next section of the test – he got the really tough ones right. It wasn't so much the final score, but the pattern in how he'd reached that score that made me wonder whether he might be malingering.

*

'Malingering' – the deliberate faking of physical or, in this case, psychiatric problems – is generally something you're more likely to come across in a personal injury compensation claim than in a forensic hospital. But malingering does have a special kind of allure to some of my more slippery customers, specifically those accused of serious crimes.

In English law, 'insanity' is a defence to any and all criminal charges. The defence can come in two forms: where the defendant claims he was insane at the time of the crime, or where the defendant asserts he is insane at the time of trial. The legal definitions and understandings of what 'insanity' might look like have morphed and mutated over centuries, in line with our understanding of the mind and human experience. In the 18th century, a person had to demonstrate the qualities of a 'wild beast or infant' to be considered insane. Since the late 19th century, courts have been concerned with 'diseases of the mind' and how these might impact a person's capacity to appreciate the effects of their actions.

There have been some notorious and well-publicized cases of malingering. American serial killers such as Ted Bundy and Kenneth Bianchi claiming murderous alter egos have penetrated the public psyche, and this may go some way to explaining why the public at large and juries in particular tend to take a cynical view of those claiming insanity as a defence – and perhaps is why it is used so rarely with any success in courts. In the UK, Soham murderer Ian Huntley is perhaps the most high-profile example of a malingerer. In the immediate days following the disappearance of the two girls he would eventually be charged with killing, Huntley gave lucid interviews to the press and actively participated in the neighbourhood's attempts to locate the girls. But when he was finally arrested and confronted with key evidence, he began staring into space, dribbling and being unresponsive. Police referred him to the high-secure Rampton Hospital for an urgent assessment of his mental state. Dr Christopher Clark, the consultant forensic psychiatrist who led the team, later said in court: 'Although Mr Huntley made clear attempts to appear insane, I have no doubt that the man currently, and at the time of the murders, was both physically and mentally sound and therefore, if he is found guilty, carried out the murders totally aware of his actions.'

Why does an offender malinger? Much of the appeal, especially to someone who has committed a crime of the magnitude of Huntley's, lies in the obvious fact that they don't have to find answers to some ignominious questions. Being considered legally insane, on the surface, may also offer an attractive option for someone seeking to evade the rigours of the law and a custodial sentence.

Except it's not that attractive because, ever since Parliament passed the Trial of Lunatics Act 1883, being deemed mad, as opposed to bad, tends to lead to a lengthy detention and treatment in a secure psychiatric institution. In the days of the asylum, that 'treatment' was likely to include beatings, being plunged into cold baths, straitjackets and even lobotomy. Today, there is a common perception that a modern-day secure hospital is the lesser of two evils, maybe even the soft option. It's undeniable that overt torture is now frowned upon and hospitals offer a more pleasant environment than prison, with an en-suite bedroom and less of the violence that exists in prisons. But they are still detention, and by no means a Club Med experience.

There's also often an assumption that admission to a secure hospital will be shorter than a prison sentence, but the truth is that people can end up staying far beyond what might have been the end of their prison term, because leaving depends on a person persuading a psychiatrist and/or Mental Health Tribunal that they have made a recovery – a nebulous concept at the best of times. A defendant deemed 'insane' can also be made subject to a hospital order with restrictions, under Sections 37 and 41 of the Mental Health Act, meaning they may be detained indefinitely, potentially forever, unless the Secretary of State for Justice decides that they can leave. Malingerers, be careful what you wish for.

*

So here was Travis with his unusual IQ test results, his coin-in-the-hand red flags and his silky backgammon skills. The other factor that piqued my interest was how he behaved in front of the consultant psychiatrist, Dr Webb, a man who at this hospital occupied the status of demigod, with a well-groomed mullet and a penchant for power dressing. It didn't seem to take Travis long to work out that the real authority didn't lie with me. As soon as he was around Dr Webb his mental state seemed to undergo a miraculous transformation and he became a textbook madman.

This was most pronounced in our weekly ward round meetings. As in any psychiatric hospital, the senior staff team in a secure unit come together for their ward rounds. These have nothing to do with physically walking around a ward in the way a doctor might in a hospital; they are resolutely static group meetings, which take place in an office, around a big table. They're usually led by the consultant psychiatrist, with an occupational therapist, a social worker, senior nurses and, at that time on the ward, me, the trainee psychologist.

In ward rounds each patient is discussed; their behaviour, mood, relationships with others and pretty much everything else analysed by the team. Medication and therapy are considered, as is any supervised leave they might get from the ward and, if it's on the cards, plans for their discharge. This overall package is called the Care Programme Approach. Patients are often invited to join meetings at the end, so they can discuss their care plans and ask permission for changes like home visits, leave or adjustments in medication.

Walking into a room full of people who you know have just been talking about you is a daunting prospect for anyone, so I always felt for them coming in. Most of us take for granted that we are the experts on our own lives and dispositions. But in this instance the patients have to defer to a team of professionals debating the inner workings of their mind and determining what is right for them. The patients often tried really hard in these meetings to mask the difficulties they were having. For many it was their only chance to see Dr Webb, who they knew wore the most important trousers and, as the only trained medical doctor in the room, prescribed their medication.

As with every team I've ever worked on, in this hospital the staff were a colourful group with no shortage of idiosyncrasies. The passive-aggressive social worker wore socks with 'fuck off' written on them, and would surreptitiously lift his trousers up at the ankles in meetings, covertly flashing the expletives on his hosiery when anyone was particularly annoying him. The occupational therapist was fastidiously hygienic, and would pass around the antibacterial gel before every meeting and wipe door handles and light switches before using them.

Privately, in fact so privately that it was only in my head, I called my supervisor Dr Renton (as in, Rent-an-opinion). He ran his own medico-legal psychology practice on the side and was proud of his growing popularity among certain lawyers who could rely upon him to identify a severe mental health issue in any or all of their clients. He would never knowingly pass up an opportunity for self-aggrandizement and had once called in sick to the hospital so that he could appear on morning television to discuss a local crime story that had attracted media interest. One of his patients came into the ward round that morning and said he'd seen Dr Renton on the television. Dr Webb, with an all-knowing sigh, made some notes. Then, looking over his glasses at the patient, said, 'Do you ever feel that the television is talking to you? Or about you? Is it broadcasting your thoughts?' It took more than a few reassurances from the occupational therapist and myself to convince Dr Webb that the exasperated patient had not been hallucinating.

There was always a certain amount of peacocking going on between Dr Renton and Dr Webb, the pair of them locked in a constant battle for status and recognition. But Renton could never quite compete with Webb who, as a psychiatrist, was always going to be higher up in the pecking order. He drove an Aston Martin V8 Vantage Le Mans – the kind of sports car that was surely compensating for something – and would sometimes let the patients sit in it long enough for a visiting relative to take a photograph.

This clinical team were not only my colleagues but a prize collection of the many strange quirks and foibles that can be found in a group of human beings at any one time, even those who are supposedly sane and functioning normally. Whatever normal is. Because, as human rights advocate Paula Caplan points out: 'normality is not "real" like a table…[it] is what psychologists call a "construct".

This means that there is no clear, real thing to which the normality label necessarily corresponds.'

One ward round morning Travis came in as usual. He was tidy and fresh as always, and sat down in the designated patient chair. The rest of us – circling the table with serious faces, like members of the Jedi Council – shuffled our papers while we waited for Dr Webb to look up from his notes and start the meeting.

Eventually he cleared his throat, welcomed Travis and asked if he knew everyone sitting round the table (he did, he had seen us all every day for the last six weeks). Travis looked around the room and said, 'I don't know.' So we went through the motions, each of us formally introducing ourselves, and Travis nodded his head and made occasional twitches and small bounces in his seat – behaviour I had never seen him exhibit before in any of the one-on-one sessions I'd had with him.

Dr Webb started to ask Travis about how he had been feeling that week, but before he had finished the sentence Travis pushed his chair back and hid his face in his hands, a picture of despondency, and then started shaking his head violently from side to side. At one point he looked to the left and jumped slightly out of his chair, as if he had been startled, all the while remaining silent.

'Are you being bothered by any voices or unusual experiences?' Dr Webb asked him. Travis repeated the question back to him, wide-eyed, as if he was having a minor religious experience. 'Bothered by hearing voices?' Then his voice lowered very slightly, and he said, 'Yes voices...really bad voices.'

Dr Webb picked up his Mont Blanc – a sure sign that something significant was coming – and Travis shifted upright in his chair (as did the rest of us in the room), like a child hoping to get a second helping of pudding.

Now waving the pen around like a small wand, Dr Webb explained to Travis that his solicitor had requested information regarding his fitness to stand trial. He launched into a well-worn, monotone speech I'd heard him deliver a few times by then: 'Fitness to plead is governed by the Criminal Procedures (Insanity and Unfitness to Plead) Act 1991. That means that we must assess whether or not you understand the charges against you.' Dr Webb raised his voice and spoke slowly for the last four words, presumably in case Travis was now also deaf and couldn't hear him.

Travis was staring straight ahead, over my shoulder, with a gormless expression on his face so drama-school perfect I had to mentally doff my cap to him for his exemplary rendering of what was once referred to as a 'lunatic', but I also noticed the capillaries in his ears turning pink. This was an indication of his blood pressure rising – and a sign that he was understanding a great deal more about the turn in the conversation than he was hoping we'd realize.

Dr Webb continued: 'And we must assess whether you understand the effect of a guilty or not guilty plea, and can instruct your legal counsel, follow evidence or challenge a juror.' Travis continued to stare past me, blinking rapidly and nodding ever so slightly with each point. Dr Webb, raising his voice again, said, 'So, Travis, can you tell me what you understand about having to go back to court soon?'

Dr Webb had lobbed the ball and now we all slowly turned our heads to see Travis's return. Travis stared at Dr Webb for a few seconds, picked up a piece of paper from the table in front of him, put a corner of it in his mouth and began to slowly chew it.

Sometimes after ward rounds, on the walk back to my shared office, I would look across the enclosed garden to what, in those less health-conscious times, was the ward's designated smoking area. I'd often see the patient we'd just been talking to go and sit on a bench in the furthest corner of the grounds to smoke. As soon as they thought they were alone and no longer being observed, they'd start to animate: nodding, gesturing, talking back to their voices. Sometimes you could see the relief on their faces, now they could finally let go. They tried so hard to maintain a veneer of sanity in the ward round.

After Travis had eaten the paper and been steered out of the meeting by a nursing assistant, I mentioned my concerns about the inconsistencies in his psychometric scores and the possibility of malingering. Travis was reporting a pretty diverse array of symptoms too – didn't it strike my colleagues as suspicious? But my comments passed with very little acknowledgement or discussion from the rest of the team. In fact it was like I hadn't said anything at all. And perhaps, because I was so keen to maintain my own outward image of the competent psychologist, I didn't challenge it in the way I would today, when I know that I am a competent psychologist. I decided that perhaps I was missing something obvious that my more experienced colleagues were seeing.

*

If I was honest, getting to the bottom of Travis and his apparent contradiction presented me with an opportunity to prove myself in this new role. Doing long hours at the hospital and finishing my master's in the evening, I was spending most of my life at work. I have no doubt that I came across as officious and superior, when in fact I was over-compensating for the fact that I was struggling quite considerably with anxiety.

After falling over at Sheffield railway station I'd continued to have attacks of severe vertigo and sickness, and had been diagnosed with Ménière's disease – a degenerative illness of the inner ear, which would eventually leave me deaf in my right ear and affect my sense of balance for good. I was learning to spot the warning signs of an attack (ringing, buzzing, humming and pain in my ears, distorted hearing, feeling off balance and like a balloon was being blown up inside my head). But the possibility of suddenly becoming dizzy and maybe dropping down here in my new role, where I was really trying to do my best professional psychologist pose, was angst provoking in itself. I couldn't tell where the anxiety ended and the Ménière's began.

If I felt an attack coming on at work, I wobbled off the ward to my office so that no one could see me breaking out in a hot sweat or trying to breathe my way through a panic attack. I would keep my head very still and walk very slowly, trying not to topple over. It probably added to the affected air I was already projecting, but I didn't want to get found out. Instead, I put all my energy into maintaining my own veneer, pretending I had everything under control. Had I been my own patient, I might even have suspected I was hiding something myself.

It became apparent that not diagnosing Travis with something would not be an option. Stark raving normal doesn't appear in any of the diagnostic manuals available to psychologists, despite the fact they contain an ever-expanding list of disorders (there are over 300 of them in the DSM alone right now, each one voted for inclusion by a committee of the world's most powerful psychiatrists, a large proportion of whom have interests in the pharmaceutical industry). Other members of the team reported that Travis had been seen 'wearing headphones and dark glasses', as if they were solely the proclivities of someone plagued by hallucinations and not something most people do when they want to listen to music in the summertime. Another colleague reported that Travis had a 'diurnal variation in mood' which meant he lived by daylight hours, went to bed early and wasn't that communicative with staff when they did their hourly checks in the evenings. It didn't sound that unusual to me – I don't like talking to people who wake me up in the middle of the night either – but as I was beginning to understand, within the context of a psychiatric ward the most banal behaviours can appear unbalanced; the lines between normal experience and 'symptoms' can become almost impossible to make out.

Which begs the question: how reliable is any psychiatric diagnosis? This was the subject of a classic experiment, conducted by the American psychologist David Rosenhan in 1973. Rosenhan sent eight ordinary people to psychiatric hospitals and told them to complain of hearing a voice – a classic diagnostic criterion of 'schizophrenia'. All eight were admitted by doctors into hospitals, and although none of them displayed any further odd behaviours or even mentioned the voice again, the majority of them received a diagnosis of a mental illness and were prescribed medication. Famously, a staff member documented evidence of one of the pseudo-patients 'engaging in writing behaviour'.

Putting pen to paper had become suspicious and loaded. Luckily for the stooges, after about three weeks most of them were declared to be in remission and discharged.

Rosenhan's experiment has been widely reported the world over. While the original study is now a bit dated, it does still serve as a useful reminder, not only of the arbitrary nature of diagnosis, but also of the way we describe and interpret behaviour though the filter of our expectations. If you're considered mad, all your behaviour is construed as madness. (Likewise, if you are considered bad, all your behaviour is construed as bad.)

*

Dr Webb diagnosed Travis with 'schizoaffective disorder', a hybrid diagnostic label describing a combination of psychotic symptoms, such as hallucinations or delusions, plus extreme highs and lows of mood. He was prescribed antipsychotic medication, not that he ever took it – because almost as soon as Travis's diagnosis was decided, he escaped.

In any kind of secure institution the windows can only ever be partially opened, as much to stop people trying to throw themselves out as to prevent them escaping. But when staff went into Travis's room one summer morning, they found he had circumvented this problem by simply removing the entire window frame, using an electric screwdriver. Subsequent investigations revealed that Travis had been having an affair with a nurse who worked night shifts at the hospital over the summer. She had brought the screwdriver in for him, along with a mobile phone so that they could talk to each other and plan his escape. This explained his 'diurnal variation in mood' and all those suspicious early nights: he had been texting his girlfriend and practising with his power tools in his room every evening (not a euphemism).

Travis was found three days later, hiding out at the nurse's house just a few miles down the road – it struck me as an unambitious escape plan, but each to their own. He didn't come back to the hospital, because in the short time that he had been missing the prosecution case against him had been dropped. This wasn't unusual; criminal cases collapse all the time. With no charges against him and – now presenting with nothing other than absolute mental clarity – he was free to go. Fortune favours the bold.

Travis never came back and, after a day or two of monumental staff gossip, he was forgotten about. But I've always remembered him. He taught me to see the people I work with as more than merely prisoners or patients, and that sanity is a spectrum, each of us differentiated by a matter of degrees. During ward rounds, while we had all been earnestly wringing our hands about what diagnostic label to give him, each of us projecting our own versions of the people we wanted to be seen as, Travis had arguably been the sanest person in the room.

The whole experience also reminded me that while faking it can be a useful strategy, at least in the short term, in the end honesty is the best policy. Discovering Travis's truth, and knowing that my early suspicions about him had been right all along, helped me begin to feel that I could trust my own judgement. Instead of pretending, it was a step towards truly becoming the psychologist I wanted to be.

CHAPTER 5
WITCHDOCTORS AND BRAINWASHERS

*I suppose it is tempting, if the only tool you have is a
hammer, to treat everything as if it were a nail.*
Abraham Maslow, *Towards a Psychology of Being*

'I reject your schizophrenia! I reject your schizophrenia!'

Marcus's deep, throaty voice boomed out from behind his door with all the force of a priest performing an exorcism. He was shouting his protests to a nurse, who was crouched down on her tiptoes, wobbling slightly as she talked to him from the other side.

I was one of three psychologists and four assistants at this secure hospital. For a place that was supposed to transform minds, it didn't exactly scream mindfulness. It was a 1960s concrete monolith, hidden way out in the sticks, down lanes and through fields, and had aged about as beautifully as the rolling hand towel contraptions, long since broken, in the staff toilets.

Beds and other furniture in secure hospital bedrooms are fixed firmly to the ground. As well as limiting the opportunities for feng shui, it means people can't blockade themselves into their rooms. But Marcus had created his own human barricade, wedging his long and slender body behind the door. As I shifted up a gear into a half-run, along the corridor towards the commotion, it occurred to me that he must have been straining every sinew he had to keep that door closed. Although his efforts were in vain; in secure hospitals, the doors are hung on hinges that open both ways.

Incoherent speech echoed around the corridor, then with clarity he shouted, 'I killed my brother! I killed him!'

This wasn't a delusion. He was right, he had. Marcus had stabbed his older brother Raymond twice in the back, lacerating his right lung and causing a fatal tension pneumothorax. It had happened outside the gates to the park, in the middle of the day, as Marcus's four-year-old daughter, still strapped into her booster seat, watched from the back of Raymond's car.

I slowed up as I got closer to the commotion, not wanting to interfere. Nurses are highly skilled and well experienced at dealing with this sort of situation and they wouldn't normally want me sticking my oar in. But it was late evening – I'd stayed on after my usual nine to five to finish writing a report – and staff numbers at this hour were lower than during the day, so I stood nearby just in case.

The nurse was holding one of those little paper cups

that looks a bit like a mini-muffin case, with pills in it. Behind her a male nursing assistant must have been anticipating trouble, as he was standing in the classic de-escalation pose: one arm loosely across his body and the other hand under his chin like *The Thinker*. The idea is that you look concerned and attentive, but your hands are in a convenient position if you need to spring into action – either through fending off an attack while protecting your face and torso, or taking hold of someone's arm or head in a physical restraint.

All mental health staff get training in the physical management of violence and aggression. Although these days the laying of hands on a patient is considered very much the last resort and the emphasis is firmly on de-escalation – calming the waters to avoid violence and confrontation. Orwell would be proud of the linguistic shift that has taken place to describe these techniques; what used to be known as 'control and restraint' is now referred to as 'care and responsibility'.

Whatever you call it, asking hard-working and undervalued hospital staff to wrestle with someone who may or may not be acting in a rational or predictable way puts most of them in an impossible position. It's no less undignified for the person being wrestled, who, already in a state of agitation, can find themselves being restrained by up to four members of staff, an experience which for anyone can be frightening and claustrophobic.

(Thankfully, I've only had to use my C&R training once; as soon as I took hold of the patient's arm, he flung himself to the floor, his arms curled in at the elbows and wrists. He was clearly an old hand at this manoeuvre. He had been in hospital for over ten years and he told me later that being restrained was the only time other human beings ever touched him.)

I didn't know the nurse crouched behind the door. She was part of the night team so our paths had not crossed before. She looked formidable, a no-nonsense matron at a boarding school. She was talking to him in a firm, uncomfortably patronizing tone.

'You were very poorly at the time,' she said, trying to persuade him to take his medication.

His response was a jumble of words and phrases: 'Don't recapture then violence brainwashers…children crying halos around my head.'

This was a 'word salad'. The term has most recently been associated with Donald Trump's more incoherent public statements, but the phrase actually originated in psychiatry, where it is used to describe a common feature of severe psychosis. Word salad is a bit like predictive text, as it conjures seemingly random and unconnected vocabulary straight out of someone's mind and sends it out of their mouths in no immediately obvious order. Although it can sound nonsensical to the listener, if you think of the words as a sort of unconventional poetry or riddle you realize that there is meaning in there, if you have the time and the patience to crack the code.

While Marcus wasn't making any real sense to me or to anyone else on the ward, it was clear that he had something important to say. And what he did manage to communicate that evening was his intense, gut-wrenching grief. He became more lucid and in a gravelly, cracked voice, he roared: 'I'm not sick. YOU are the ones that are sick in the head!' His distress was now audibly escalating. 'I killed my brother! Because of you!'

The nurse replied, 'No Marcus, it was because you have an illness and that's why I want to give you this medication. It will help you feel better.'

'Get out of my house. I reject your schizophrenia.' He was getting louder and more forceful as this fruitless exchange developed. Although they were speaking the same language, they may as well have been from different planets. Marcus was getting angry because he felt he wasn't being heard, while the well-meaning but old-school nurse seemed oblivious.

The nursing assistant and I exchanged glances, a little voltage of mutual understanding passing between us, and I let him know I was going to step in. I gave the nurse a wave and pushed my hand downwards in the air, to signal she needed to take it down a notch. But she didn't know who I was and seemed to look through me. She ploughed on regardless.

I sensed that the situation was escalating and felt like it was time to intervene. I stepped forward. 'Marcus, it's Kerry.'

He shouted back, 'Witchdoctor! Witchdoctors and brainwashers.'

The nurse looked at me and opened her mouth, as if to shut the conversation down. Before she had a chance to intervene, I tried my luck.

'Marcus, I can hear that you are feeling really frustrated. Tell me about what's happening.'

Everything went quiet.

'I killed my brother,' Marcus said.

'Yes, yes you did, you killed your brother.'

The nurse stood up and took a step back, her lips pursed so tightly they had almost disappeared. I suggested, as tactfully as I could, that she could perhaps give us some time to talk and maybe pop back in 15 minutes.

And then I sat with Marcus for a bit, listening to him speak. The door was ajar, and I sat opposite him, saying very little but attempting to make sense of what he had to tell me. Sometimes you just have to sit with a person, validate what they are feeling and not be afraid of their pain and grief. Marcus had done something dreadful and irreversible. The kind of thing that can't simply be blithely explained or medicated away.

After Marcus had offloaded for a while, the nurse returned and silently passed him some tablets and a glass of water before departing. I didn't see her again until I left that night, and when I said goodbye she didn't reply.

*

On the day he killed his brother, Marcus believed that Raymond was possessed by demons.

Marcus had been haunted by graphic visions of Raymond beating him for weeks. These fleeting but vivid images were agonizing for Marcus and, in his state of mind, he believed that they had been deliberately placed inside his head to punish him. Malevolent voices in his head claimed that they had a hold over Raymond, that they were torturing him and it was all Marcus's fault. In among the battle noise and chaos in his mind, only one clear thought emerged: he had to kill his sibling.

After his arrest, Marcus had been diagnosed with 'schizophrenia'. Schizophrenia is, like so many of our diagnoses, a catch-all term for a plethora of altered states. This includes everything from hallucinations (seeing, hearing, feeling or smelling things), delusions (believing paranoid or extraordinary things) and muddled thinking to difficulties concentrating or a lack of emotion and drive.

It is one of the profession's most broad and diversely applied labels and has expanded and altered further and wider over time. Unfortunately 'schizophrenia' has now become a derogatory and often insulting moniker that leaves little room for nuance or individuality under its gloomy and heavy-duty stamp. It is a condition that everyone thinks they understand, a common trope and easy punchline in popular culture. You are never alone with schizophrenia, so the old joke goes. Or as Billy Connolly put it: 'Roses are red, violets are blue, I'm a schizophrenic and so am I.'

The common understanding of schizophrenia means Norman Bates, Jekyll and Hyde, the Mad Hatter. Calling someone a 'schizo' is now shorthand for someone who loses their temper easily, or appears to be like a different person when they are enraged. But that's not schizophrenia, that's being angry.

It has also come to be associated with dangerous, violent or criminal behaviour; horror films are full of apparently psychotic axe-wielding maniacs. A 2012 study of the representation of schizophrenia in Hollywood looked at 40 films featuring characters with that diagnosis released between 1990 and 2010. It found that over 80 per cent of them displayed violent behaviour and nearly a third committed homicides.

And it's not just the fictional world – violent crime is the most frequent and pervasive theme in coverage of schizophrenia stories in the news.

But the stereotypes fall down when you consider that 1 per cent of the world's population has been given a diagnosis of schizophrenia, giving us around 51 million schizophrenic people worldwide. If all of these people were violently assaulting and killing others we'd be stepping over the corpses in the street.

In fact, there are between 50 and 70 cases of homicide a year in the UK involving those, like Marcus, who have a severe mental health problem at the time of killing. Of course, this is still far too many and preventing these tragedies should be a concern for everyone. But most of the over 220,000 people in the UK with a diagnosis of schizophrenia live unremarkable, peaceful lives. They are ordinary people in your street, your office and your local pub, posing no threat or danger to anyone. But their stories don't sell newspapers, so you, like me, only come into contact with the horror stories.

So what makes some people with a diagnosis of schizophrenia pose a risk while others don't? Research tells us that the answer lies in the many other factors that make up human existence. The risk of violent behaviour is typically linked to other circumstances, problems or issues which are not necessarily directly connected to someone's mental ill-health. In particular this includes substance misuse but also a fundamental lack of personal and/or professional support and a previous history of violence, either as the victim or the perpetrator. However, contrary to the media headlines, the rate of violence in those who have been diagnosed with schizophrenia, while marginally above the rate in those who haven't, is still too slight to be able to predict with any precision.

*

This was just after the turn of the millennium, and there was a steadily increasing demand for beds in secure hospitals. One look at the NHS England balance sheets at the time told you the story: early intervention, community and mental health crisis services were not receiving nearly the same level of funding and investment as secure services. In fact expenditure on medium- and high-secure mental health services made up around one-fifth of all public spending on adult mental health care at the time. The money was being spent on detention rather than prevention, the horses had bolted long before any doors were being locked.

And whereas I had once been almost the only forensic psychologist in the village, more and more forensic psychologists were moving into secure hospitals, many from the prison service, from where they brought a certain philosophy and model of intervention with them.

The fashion was (and still is) for treatment programmes tightly packaged into step-by-step manuals and delivered to patients in groups: Sex Offender Treatment Group, Fire-setters Group, Anger Management Group, and so on. Each combines a series of educational and CBT-based sessions aimed at teaching participants the new attitudes, values, beliefs and patterns of behaviour they will need as reformed citizens. Delivered with dogmatic methodology, these programmes are administered by psychologists – but also often by other staff, in truth by anyone with a manual and a few days' training. It is psychological practice industrialized – with your programme sheets, scripts and questionnaires in front of you, you write reports using templates, you rate engagement on a scale, you tick boxes to show rigid procedure has been adhered to. It's prescriptive for everyone involved – patients were never in straitjackets, but it increasingly felt as though you, the psychologist, were.

I am an advocate of cognitive behavioural therapy and other derived therapies for treating a whole range of problems, such as phobias and mood issues. But their effectiveness in preventing reoffending in the long term is still up for debate – no matter how fervent somebody's professed changes in attitudes and beliefs in the artificial environment of a prison or secure hospital, whether it will have the desired effect on their behaviour many years into the future when they are in the real world isn't clear. While my feelings about the usefulness of these one-size-fits-all group sessions were conflicted at best, I was left feeling certain that they trained many patients to become skilled at saying what they thought their Stepford psychologist wanted to hear.

Not Marcus though. His frequent refrain of 'I reject your schizophrenia' was becoming the soundtrack to an impasse at his every ward round. Meetings that usually culminated in Marcus pointing at us – the senior staff – and calling us 'witchdoctors and brainwashers'.

Despite being prescribed large doses of antipsychotic medication, which he always grudgingly accepted, he continued to be tormented by voices. He could often be overheard having intense, irate discussions while alone in his bedroom. His risk assessment made for hair-raising and pessimistic reading, describing him as 'paranoid, treatment resistant and lacking insight'.

Marcus faced another, more insidious problem too, something that might have been unconsciously threaded into our ongoing assessment of his high risk of violence. Because not only was Marcus loud and non-conformist, he was black.

In 2002, not long before Marcus came to the hospital, the Bennett Inquiry had been commissioned. It followed the death of David Bennett, an African-Caribbean man, who died after being restrained by staff at a medium-secure unit. The report found that black men were generally regarded by staff in psychiatric hospitals as 'more aggressive, more alarming, more dangerous and more difficult to treat' and that they tended to receive higher doses of medication than white people given similar diagnoses. It concluded that people from black and minority ethnic communities were six times more likely to be sectioned, more likely to stay longer as in-patients in psychiatric wards, and more likely to be prescribed medication or electroconvulsive therapy instead of psychological treatment or 'talking therapies'.

In short, the UK's mental health services are riddled with racial discrimination. I had seen plenty of blatant, in-your-face racism in prisons, but it is altogether more surreptitious in the psychiatric hospital setting. Marcus's mistrust of us was perhaps not as irrational as it appeared.

He grew up in Birmingham, as part of a second-generation Jamaican-British family, his father arriving in the 1960s as part of the Windrush Generation. Hostility to black people was still overt, even socially acceptable. His father found a job as a taxi driver, but wasn't permitted to enter the pubs he drove his customers to and from. Signs saying 'No coloureds' or 'No West Indians' were commonplace. Just a few years earlier, Conservative MP Peter Griffiths had won a local election in nearby Smethwick with the slogan 'If you want a n****r for a neighbour, vote Labour'. In fact the racism in the area was so virulent that the US political activist Malcolm X went to Smethwick in 1965. He was shot dead in New York just nine days after his visit.

Marcus told the story of how one day his dad decided to go into the pub, regardless, and family legend was that, for a short time, a sign saying 'No blacks, No Irish, No dogs' which he took home from it, became the centrepiece of the kitchen at home.

This pathos-heavy scene was about as good as

home life got for Marcus. His much-loved father died when he was six and he lived in a one-bedroom flat with his mother and brother, and occasionally also his grandmother, for the next ten years.

Marcus described himself as a skinny, timid child, overshadowed by his bigger, older and more charismatic brother. He told me that his grandmother was a fearsome woman who was devoutly and extremely Pentecostal. She believed in witchcraft and possession by evil spirits. When one winter a leak had begun to let rainwater in through the wall of the flat's kitchen, his grandmother had declared it the work of the devil in Marcus. He recounted how she had made Raymond hold him down on the kitchen table while she beat him on the back with a leather belt to expunge his 'wickedness'. Marcus said that when his mother eventually intervened, it was one of the few times he had seen her stand up to his grandmother.

With this cultural context in mind, Marcus's references to 'witchdoctors' suddenly made far more sense. And while we were certainly not witchdoctors (no chicken's blood here, although with our insistence on variably effective medications and magic formula therapy manuals, I could see where he was coming from), the esteem in which he held medical doctors might not have been much higher.

*

I was in a room with Marcus, the air thick with boredom as we prepared to get through the upcoming hour that was the Mental Health Awareness Group.

Together with a psychology assistant, we were here with six other patients, most of them fairly new admissions to the hospital, but not necessarily new to this experience. The gloomy mood was matched by the room, a shabby basement with high windows around the top, like holes in a deep pocket.

Channelling the spirit of a middle manager on a team bonding retreat, the psychology assistant pulled back the cover of a flip-chart and invited everyone to name all the different symptoms of psychiatric illnesses. The thinking behind this exercise was to help the patients connect their more unusual experiences to recognized symptoms. Thereby encouraging a light-bulb moment where the group members recognize that they have a medical issue and are persuaded to embrace their diagnostic label and follow the recommended course of treatment. Voila! This is what psychiatry prizes as 'insight'.

Although we had a few slender contributions ('not sleeping', 'thinking your food is contaminated', 'feeling sad' and 'saying that you are Jesus, even when you really aren't Jesus'), most of the group sat stony faced, despite the assistant's artistry with the flip chart and marker pen. They were there for the biscuits, and to pass the time until lunch.

Apart from Marcus, who was very engaged, but not quite in the way that we wanted. With every answer we extracted from the listless group, he would tut loudly, suck his teeth and mutter under his breath. He would fidget around, crossing and uncrossing his arms and shifting around in his chair. And yet, he was paying close attention.

A couple of times I heard him mumble: 'They're telling us we are sick in the head…'

When you have one particularly distracting group member like this, it often helps to give them a job to do, to keep them occupied and to minimize the disruption to the rest of the group.

I invited Marcus up to the front so he could write up the words on the flip chart as the others did – or didn't – shout them out.

He leapt up and strode to the front, grabbed the felt marker pen from the assistant's hand and scribbled in giant letters:

PAIN

'All of this shit is pain…just pain is all,' he said, waving the marker across the flip chart like a university lecturer who had just revealed the answer to a complex equation. Then, addressing the group members, 'Don't let these brainwashers tell you that you are sick.'

The room was silent, as everyone quickly considered whether he'd just said something mind blowing or was talking utter nonsense.

This wasn't the textbook Mental Health Awareness Group answer (and, of course, the psychology assistant and I were working from a thick textbook, with accompanying illustrated handouts for all group participants), but it was very hard to deny the truth of Marcus's response. Because his life had been undoubtedly painful, and all of the 'symptoms' that the group had outlined were indeed just examples of what can happen when people suffer.

Immediately after this fleeting moment of existential clarity from Marcus, the assistant thanked him for his help and ushered him to sit down. Which he did, with his arms folded once more and his eyes tightly shut. We'd had a brief opportunity to connect with him and we'd missed it.

While the earth didn't seem to move for anyone else in the room, that session was groundbreaking for me. It brought into dazzling focus the misgivings I'd been harbouring for some time.

*

There is a growing queue of well-intentioned celebrities lining up to tell us that mental distress is an 'illness just like any other', and that we should seek help for our broken minds in the same way as we would a broken leg. While being open as a society and ready to discuss mental health problems is a positive thing, the evidence that mental 'illness' can be tested for, diagnosed and treated with the same certainty as a physical disease is far from conclusive.

With a physical illness, having a diagnosis can be a relief – finally knowing what is causing your symptoms and being able to put a name to it means that you know what you're dealing with and may even be on the way to recovering. In the same way, being given a psychiatric diagnosis is helpful for some people – it acknowledges the real difficulties that people experience and can allow them to obtain the help and support they need. But for a lot of others, having their mental health problems described as 'illnesses' feels oppressive.

The components of what we tend to think of as an illness can be restrictive – it's typically something that we can catch, something caused by diseases, something that can be cured, something that is wrong with us. But many mental health issues simply don't share these characteristics. Referring to mental illness suggests that a mental health problem is qualitatively different from your garden-variety emotional pain or confusion, and results from an underlying brain disease. It negates the fact that psychological distress, in whatever form it is exhibited/plays out, is frequently a plausible reaction to the slings and arrows that life throws at us.

Some diagnostic labels are easier to swallow than others. 'Anxiety disorder' or 'depressive disorder', for example, don't tend to carry such negative associations in the public mind as 'schizophrenia'. As psychologist and former psychiatric patient Dr Jay Watts puts it, 'Yes, there is stigma, but not the rampant sticky, staining discrimination one gets with diagnoses associated with serious mental illness.' As a result of this prejudice, for someone experiencing phenomena such as hearing voices, or being convinced of things that others find bizarre, their psychological distress is often as much a result of facing people's reactions to their experiences as of the experiences themselves.

There is evidence that purely physical causes are more at play with some diagnostic categories than with others. For example, there is some evidence for neurobiological underpinnings to 'bipolar disorder', yet, for a great many people, the anguish that leads them to seek professional help has far clearer established links to social disadvantage: poverty, poor housing, insecure and low-paid jobs, missing out on formal education, living in stressful environments or having to move home frequently. Problems that may be difficult for others to understand (believing that you are Jesus, for example) are often related to stressful events and life circumstances, particularly abuse or other forms of trauma. Between half and three-quarters of people receiving mental health care report having been either physically or sexually abused as children. In short, mental distress is more likely a product of complex, overlapping personal and social factors than simply wonky brain chemistry or unfortunate genetics.

Being given a diagnosis can be both a positive and a negative thing, so what is the best thing to do? A frequent response from professionals and service users involved in debating the issue is that people should be free to choose how, or if, to name and make sense of their experience. Certainly, in Marcus's case, he was unwilling to accept the illness explanation that he was being force-fed. Yet he had killed somebody. And that's what got me thinking – did that mean he had forfeited the right to choose whether or not to accept his diagnostic label?

*

Luckily for both of us, there was no Fratricide Group on the hospital curriculum. I began to have one-to-one sessions with Marcus and never referred to 'schizophrenia', or used any other medical language in front of him again.

We met twice a week, in a small consulting room on the main ward (at least until a directive came through that all patients, regardless of need, must be offered individual time with a psychologist of one hour a week – no more, no less – to meet audit requirements). No longer stuck in a perpetual deadlock over what was 'wrong' with him, we started piecing together and making sense of what had happened to him.

The young Marcus had left home as soon as he could,

moving in with his girlfriend, who he'd met at a lively cafe that he used to visit at lunchtimes and after work. The pair, both just 20, had a daughter together, and Marcus said it was soon after her first birthday that he began to hear voices.

Many of us will have auditory hallucinations at some point in our lives. Hearing your name being called when there is no one around, or someone speak just as you are drifting off to sleep, is a common enough experience. In one small study of British mental health nurses, 83 per cent described at least once having heard a voice 'as if someone had spoken aloud rather than a thought or feeling'. Hearing the voice of a deceased loved one is often reported by those who are recently bereaved, and is mostly described as a comforting, rather than upsetting, phenomenon.

I experienced something fundamentally similar to voice-hearing during my own stressful times, hearing the telephone ringing when it hadn't. The first and second time it happened, I picked up my telephone to nothing but the dial tone. The third time it happened, I thought that perhaps it was time to book myself a holiday. After that, it didn't happen again.

When Marcus started hearing a female voice, commenting about what he was doing when he was at home alone one evening, he thought little of it at first. But she became more frequent, more critical. She made comments about how his car was dirty. Minor nagging at first, but then calling him lazy, useless. Hearing this so clearly but with no physical human in the room to attribute it to, he searched for the most reasonable explanation, coming to the conclusion that, as she was the only woman he lived with, it must surely be his girlfriend who was somehow behind it.

He started to hear the voice even when he was away from the house, and she was gradually joined by a chorus of others, all talking at the same time. He began to shout at them – 'Why are you doing this to me?' 'Are you spying on me?' 'Leave me alone!' – but they were louder, stronger and more confident than he was. More voices joined in; some were less hostile, friendly even, and he said he felt they were supportive and useful to him. Some were funny and made him laugh, they sang nursery rhymes to him that his girlfriend sang to their daughter, and talked back to him if he 'thought' in response to them.

Having satisfied himself *who* was behind the voices, Marcus described how he turned his attention to the questions of *how* and *why*. The only plausible explanation that he could come up with was that his girlfriend was unhappy in their relationship and was practising witchcraft on him – a conclusion that isn't so out of left field when we remember his grandmother's beliefs.

I have seen plenty of unusual belief systems in this job.

If someone feels that external forces are controlling their mind or body, it often starts to make sense to them when they attribute it to something religious or supernatural. Another common possessive experience is aliens, who like to beam thoughts via radioactive light waves into the carrier's brain (arguably at least as plausible as gods and demons – if not more so. It all depends on your unique way of looking at the world).

Marcus confronted his girlfriend, angry at what he saw as her attempts to control him, but also terrified by what was happening. With their young daughter in the flat, his girlfriend was frightened by his odd behaviour and threw him out. He couldn't go back to his mother and grandmother, with whom he'd had very little contact since he left, so with nowhere else to go he began to sleep in his car. It was the start of a sustained period of misery and rejection for Marcus, who, it seemed to him, no one wanted to be around.

Just a few weeks after becoming homeless, he was fired from his job. And he had been particularly upset one day when he was thrown out of the cafe where he had been a regular for years. He shifted in his seat and hit the arm of his chair defiantly with his outstretched palm as he told me how the boyfriend of one of the owners had come over to him and told him he needed to get out because he was 'talking to himself and freaking everyone out'. He came back to that story a few times; it had obviously been a nail in his coffin, seeing it as proof that, as he put it, he had been cursed.

I could imagine Marcus openly talking to voices no one else could hear, wandering the streets at midday when the rest of the world was busy working. He had become the guy you cross the street to avoid. When he told me about his ejection from the cafe, I couldn't help but think about the parallels with his father's experience of being denied entry to the pub, all those years before.

With his living conditions worsening, the critical voices in his mind became stronger and more forceful. He'd begun self-medicating with cannabis, 'to get some peace from it', he explained. But it had only made things worse. Marcus had stayed in touch with his older brother, Raymond, who had a family of his own and lived close by. Raymond agreed to facilitate contact between Marcus and his daughter, being present during the short trips to the park and occasionally the cinema, which his ex-girlfriend permitted on the condition that Raymond stayed with them. Hearing of his drug use, however, his ex-girlfriend denied him access to his daughter, and, in a double blow, Raymond's wife would no longer allow Marcus in their house because he made her uncomfortable.

He had lost his home, his job and the only people he had to rely on. When he talked about this period he kept returning to the cafe, a place where he'd once been so welcome, and how he'd been told not to come back. The critical voices were telling him he was bad and wicked, words that seemed to echo his grandmother's criticisms of him as a child, and felt all the more onerous as a result.

As Marcus began to explain what his voices had begun to tell him, I saw how the story had come to its sorry end. The voices started telling him to hurt himself. He scratched himself on his arms until he bled, hit his head on a brick wall – the voices bickering over who was in charge and what he should do next. As his external life became more difficult and unhappy, so his voices became more shrill and urgent. He described feeling how the voices were by now so much more powerful than he was that he knew he would never be able to ignore them, or defy them.

To the excluded Marcus, Raymond began to emerge as the focal point of all his worries.

Feeling that life was spiralling out of control at a faster pace than he could cope with, he described how his hallucinations were responsible for 'brainwashing' him into believing that all his misfortune was because of his brother, and that Marcus needed to eliminate him. They described how Raymond was possessed, and being tortured by, demons that were cursing Marcus and causing all of his unhappiness. Marcus decided that it was now his task to kill Raymond, therefore killing the evil spirit that had possessed him, and in doing so reclaim his family.

He readily admitted that he planned how he would do it. He described arranging to meet Raymond before going into a hardware shop and stealing a knife. A series of rational acts within an irrational story. He was quite right when he said: 'I knew I was killing him.'

*

I hadn't realized it at the time, but Marcus accusing us of being 'brainwashers and witchdoctors' was the beginning of his recovery.

'Social rank theory' argues that our feelings and emotions are notably influenced by how we see ourselves fitting into the social pecking order – particularly the extent to which we feel inferior to, and looked down on by, other people. This can result in believing and doing 'what we're told', even when the voices telling us what to do are inside our own heads. When Marcus killed Raymond, he was at rock bottom, seeing himself as the lowest of the low. Maybe this was why he was particularly susceptible to obeying, rather than questioning, challenging and resisting, the commands from the voices.

Refusing to accept his diagnostic label showed that he was beginning to challenge the credibility of what he was hearing from authority figures (albeit real ones, in this case), rather than just going along with what he was instructed to believe. A much safer way for Marcus to be, in my opinion. Yet there was more to it than that. By refusing to accept that he had an illness, he was also facing up to the choice he had made to kill Raymond.

I worked with Marcus for over a year but moved on from the hospital before he did. I bumped into him again many years later, when I was visiting a low-secure hospital. He worked in its small on-site cafe. He had put on a bit of weight and I almost didn't recognize him until he waved and shouted, 'It's the witchdoctor!', and I was left in no doubt. He told me that he was starting to take small steps towards rebuilding relationships with his mother and daughter, who visited him there. And he had taken on an unofficial role as patient-mentor, running mindfulness groups. In fact, he had become something of a mindfulness maestro. He still heard voices, he explained, but he could ignore them now, even 'shush them up' if he wanted to.

If Marcus had learned to challenge his voices, I had also begun to think differently about the way I approached my patients, and to open up new conversations around mental health. Conversations that go beyond the usual 'illness' script and respect the person's own construction of their history and experience, whatever words they use to describe it. Working with him made me wonder: if we could see people who act in strange or hard to understand ways, as Marcus had that day in Mental

Health Awareness Group, as simply others in pain, rather than paint them with the stigma of a disorder, would we all be more willing and able to reach out to them? And would tragedies like Raymond's death be more easily avoided?

CHAPTER 6
POWER PLAYS

The quest to understand violence has led me
to view a criminal's actions as the shadows cast
by his own inner narratives.
Professor David Canter, *Criminal Shadows*

The day I took the call from the police asking for my help with an investigation, a double-height mesh fence was being put up right outside my office and the noise had given me a headache.

I was working in a secure hospital at the time, and the fence was going up because of a patient who had escaped a few weeks earlier and become the subject of what must have been the slowest police chase of 2003, if not in history. He'd managed to walk straight out of the grounds and had stolen a tractor that somehow still had the keys in it. Police didn't actually need to chase him at all, they just parked their car at the gate to the field and probably had time to complete a crossword as they waited for him to get to them.

Despite this event being the opposite of dramatic, the local press had gone large with fear-mongering headlines about an escaped madman on the loose. So the hospital spent thousands on ramping up some of the more visible security, reassuring our genteel neighbours in this well-to-do rural area that all was under control. They put in an electric barrier, so that every car had to stop on its way in, and employed a former nursing assistant, 'Big Nathan', as a security guard. He seized this new power with both hands, and wouldn't let you in without correct ID even if he knew you. Even the therapy dog, a shih-tzu called Larry, didn't make it in to work one morning because he didn't have photo ID.

The patient who had briefly escaped had learning disabilities and had been convicted of several arson attacks. He had a habit of climbing over the dark green fence that separated the outside courtyard of his ward from the main grounds. He would usually return to the front of the ward and wave at the intercom camera to get back in. He once buzzed through asking for a plaster, because he'd cut his finger on the chain-link fence during his climb.

He acted this way because he wanted us to know that he could. And sometimes because he had a problem that he felt he couldn't solve. It was a plea for help – he wanted us to know that he needed help figuring out what to do.

*

I've never considered myself to be a 'profiler' – for one thing, it's not a real job – but people seem to like calling me a profiler. And I'll take it, because it makes me sound far more exotic than the tea-drinking northerner that I am, as if I possess magical powers. Thanks to TV's depiction of forensic psychologists (in particular *Criminal Minds* and *Wire In The Blood*), the criminal profiler has acquired a status in the collective consciousness as someone who is brilliant but eccentric, someone able to divine the exact identity of a hitherto unknown killer from a few cryptic clues, a quick cigarette at a crime scene and a lot of thin air.

But it's not like that in real life. So-called profilers are in fact ordinary human beings, who do not possess any wizarding genes whatsoever. What they can do is bring a fresh eye, and apply some psychological knowledge, to the existing evidence and/or suspects in a case. Profilers are brought in as consultants by the police when they need a different perspective on an investigation, or a new way to access information they know they haven't yet discovered. They might help link a series of crimes, plan interviews, perhaps help the police understand how personality and mental state could drive an offender's behaviour or affect a victim's recollection of events. Only rarely is a psychologist brought in to determine a 'profile', a list of the likely personality, history and lifestyle characteristics of an unknown offender, inferred from an examination of the crime and where it took place. And the notion of a lone clinical Columbo tracking serial killers really only exists in the imagination of filmmakers. Not least because UK criminologists estimate that a maximum of four serial killers are operating in this country at any given time (which is fairly good news or utterly terrifying, depending on your point of view).

The whole area of applying psychology to the process of catching criminals and bringing them to justice is now known as 'investigative psychology' and during my career it has blossomed into its own distinct discipline, with dedicated university courses, specially trained police officers and sophisticated databases of information and software. The discipline has broadened into a whole range of investigative areas, contributing to everything from detecting tax evasion to interpreting terrorist threats. Perhaps the question I get asked most by students is: how do I become a profiler? I tell them to study and become an academic, or join the police force and do the training in investigative psychology. Then privately I think that if they haven't managed to investigate that for themselves, they might have to up their game.

*

I also sometimes give them a dose of realism about profiling, using an analogy about the time I skived off school with my first boyfriend, Jamie Rabourn. In our 16-year-old wisdom we decided our time that sunny day would be much better spent lazing around in the long grass behind our school than it would in a boring classroom.

I got home later on and Mum asked me how my day had been. Leaning breezily into my deception I replied, 'Oh OK, a bit boring, just the usual.'

Without even raising an eyebrow she replied, 'That's funny, because it looks to me a lot like you spent the afternoon lazing in the long grass with Jamie Rabourn.'

How could she possibly know that? I demanded to know. She said, victorious: 'Because I'm your mother.' In that moment I felt sure she was not only my mother, but a woman with super-human powers of perception and deduction.

Actually, she'd received a phone call from school telling her I had disappeared after morning roll-call, and coincidentally so had Jamie Rabourn. I noticed later that evening that I also had lots of long grass still lodged in my hair. Marvellous as she is, my mum doesn't possess precognitive skills. She had narrowed down the options based on the evidence, the most likely probabilities and her hard-won understanding of teenage behaviour and motivations.

*

I had been part of the well-established psychology team at this secure hospital for a year but I did a three-day week now, while beginning to build my private practice part-time, teaching post-grads applied forensic psychology at Manchester University and acting as an expert witness in court.

I didn't usually spend much time in my office anyway, but I'd been purposefully avoiding it because of the noise of the heavy-duty power tools on full blast. It was lucky that I was even at my desk when the phone rang that day.

Keen to escape the din, I snatched up the receiver. It was Detective Sergeant Steve Allbright, an interview coordinator from the Serious Crime Review Team. He was looking for a psychologist to help with a murder investigation: he had a crime and a prime suspect but not enough evidence to charge him. A first round of interviews hadn't borne any fruit and they'd like some help with the next round. Could I help?

I explained that I didn't have any hands-on experience in this kind of exercise, but he said it didn't matter, he just needed a psychologist's view. There was unlikely to be any pay in it, but could I be tempted? It turns out that when a police officer calls and asks for your help in a murder investigation, even if it is pro bono and you've never done it before, you say yes.

*

At the police station, Steve showed me to the office he shared with the rest of the team. There was a familiar feeling of organized chaos, with piles of paperwork everywhere and the air ripe with coffee and microwaved lunches. I had powdered milk in my tea and it looked like rusty water.

Steve presented the facts of the story: a 62-year-old

man, Malcolm Johns, had been murdered in his home seven years ago – killed in his bed, while his wife slept next door in the second bedroom. Police had never found his killer.

Around the same time, there had been a spate of burglaries in the area where Johns had lived – a sprawling post-war council estate of mainly terraced houses, each with a small front and back garden. All the burglaries had a similar modus operandi, with nothing too unusual about it: entry was made through a back door and the usual household small electrics, jewellery and other valuables had been taken. But, more unusually, the burglar had entered the house in the middle of the night.

If you believe TV and film writers, burglaries take place when everyone is sound asleep as the burglar plans to sneak through a window undetected. In reality, most burglars don't want to come into contact with other people (in convict slang, those who do burgle by night are known as 'creepers') – the majority of break-ins to homes take place during the day while people are at work and their houses are empty. Burglary traffic hits its peak in the late afternoons of early winter, when it is dark enough to provide intruders with cover, but still not time for most people to be home from work.

A young data analyst, Jo, joined us. She was new to the force and had a special interest in crime scene analysis and geographical profiling – analysis of the location(s) connected to a crime that can help identify where the offender is likely to live and narrow down a pool of suspects. She had been recruited in anticipation of the roll-out of HOLMES2, an information technology system that holds masses of information about major crime incidents and allows cross referencing from every force in the country, which is now used by all UK police forces. But hi-tech HOLMES2 hadn't quite arrived yet, so she had been doing things the old-fashioned way. She had spent days overlaying a map with acetate and putting fine felt-tip dots where night-time burglaries had taken place over a one-year period either side of the murder. But her labours amounted to an indecipherable mass of tiny red dots, far too condensed and numerous to reveal any pattern.

A number of burglary victims in this group had reported not only the theft of items from their homes, but also waking up to see a man wearing a balaclava standing at the end of their bed. If they were unfortunate enough to wake up to this terrifying spectre, the man had barked the same order at them to turn over, face down, and put their hands behind their head. He had then stood silently watching them for a while – some said moments, for others it was minutes – before he eventually disappeared. None of the victims could identify any of the man's facial features; recall of faces is poor at the best of times, and pretty much impossible in a dark room when a balaclava is involved. Other physical characteristics they reported were variable; his accent was possibly local, nondescript. But all the witnesses told police the same thing – there was silence in the room, save for the sound of their own heavy breathing. He didn't seem to do anything. He just watched them for a while and left.

Jo had put these specific incidents onto a separate sheet of acetate and they were much easier to see – about 19 little red dots that formed a thin corridor, roughly half a mile by four miles. The burglar had gone on a shopping spree and this red corridor was his high street. There were just a couple of outliers, burglaries that had taken place around the time of Malcolm Johns' murder, but in locations slightly further afield than the burglar's preferred area. If the cases were linked – and that was still an assumption – it looked like the old man's death had rattled the perpetrator enough to drive him temporarily from his usual beat.

Another crime that had taken place in the area, at a storage facility on an industrial estate that backed onto the residential neighbourhood, had played out very differently. As Steve told me about this crime, Jo carefully added a blue dot to one end of the existing passage of red.

Eight months after Malcolm Johns had been killed, two teenage boys and their parents were in one of the lock-ups on a Saturday afternoon, sorting through boxes full of their recently deceased grandmother's belongings. As the four of them were busy rummaging and boxing up, a man wearing a balaclava and holding what looked like a gun (it turned out to be an imitation Browning MK2 pistol – police will still treat it as a real firearm if you start waving one around) stepped calmly inside the unit and ushered them all to stand facing the wall and put their hands behind their heads, firing-squad style. As Steve and Jo told me this, I raised an eyebrow at the audacity of it: keeping four people under control in an unpredictable, semi-public space is no mean undertaking. Even with a convincing-looking weapon, you still have the threat of someone deciding to challenge you.

The robber kept the four of them facing the wall, with their hands behind their heads. They described how he rifled casually through their belongings and loaded his bag. Then, still very much at his leisure, he walked up behind the mother, who was standing at the far end of the line, and ran his hands over her breasts. Still standing behind her, he then put his hand down the front of her trousers. A sexual assault. He took his hand away and stood behind the family for a few moments longer, then slipped out of the lock-up.

Nothing on the storage warehouse CCTV showed the robber leaving the facility. But police were eventually able to identify and arrest a local man, Ian

Hogan, a former member of staff at the storage unit, who still rented his own lock-up there. He hadn't been seen leaving the place because he hadn't left it. He'd gone straight into his own lock-up and stayed there for some time, knowing exactly where the CCTV cameras were positioned, when staff rotated and how he could emerge without drawing attention to himself.

Hogan – in his 30s, now unemployed and married with two young sons – lived just outside the residential estate. Jo dabbed a second blue dot on the acetate, and the red line was now perfectly sandwiched between the two blue markers: Hogan's home at one end and the storage facility at the other. It wasn't a geographical profiler's dream – serial offences more typically fall within a rough circle, around the central point of an offender's home – but it was a significant pattern.

Hogan was convicted of aggravated robbery for the storage warehouse offence but, for reasons best known to the Crown Prosecution Service, he had not been separately charged with the sexual assault. He had served nearly half his seven-year sentence and would soon be on his way back home. He had also been linked to some of the night-time burglaries, the number of which had plummeted in the area since his move to prison. Linked, because it wasn't possible to conclusively prove that he was the creeper, even though many of the stolen items were now living happily in his storage unit. In fact, the unit was heaving with valuable goods: televisions and electricals, jewellery, tools, replica and antique weapons. There were also plenty of seemingly worthless, mundane things: calendars, hairbrushes, draught excluders. Hogan admitted nothing, claiming that he acquired much of the lock-up's contents from men he traded with in the pub.

Of particular significance among the jumble of items found at Hogan's lock-up was a watch belonging to Malcolm Johns – a 1970s watch with a gold face and a worn-in brown leather strap. It was the kind of watch that might have had sentimental value, but wasn't worth much money. Like all the other items, Hogan insisted he'd bought it from a stranger in the pub and no one could prove otherwise.

*

The serial offender's habit of keeping 'trophies' has long been a favourite with novelists and scriptwriters; the more gruesome the trinket or in some cases body part, the better. But they don't only exist in crime fiction. In 2006 the so-called 'shoe rapist' James Lloyd from Rotherham was found to have kept over a hundred pairs of shoes behind a trap door at his office, all of them taken from his victims after he had attacked them.

Why do some criminals need a souvenir? A trophy doesn't have to be a fetish item. Even the most mundane of objects can act as a form of proof, a physical anchor to their crime, and all the psychological meaning attached to it. In the case of a sexual assault or murder, holding it allows them to relive the excitement and stimulation, to be able to access the fantasy at any time, over and over again. I have even known some offenders make gifts of their trophy items, covertly reasserting their dominance and control over a different person – the secret knowledge that they could do to them what they did to their victim, if they so choose.

*

In addition to the discovery of the watch, Steve explained that a partial shoe print had been found at the scene of the break-in at the Johns' home, in Hogan's size. It was however from the sole of a very common trainer, and no matching shoes had been found at Hogan's lock-up or home. There were some black wool fibres (possibly from gloves or a balaclava) on Johns' body, matching the fibres found at the back-door entry point of one of the 'hands-on-head' burglaries, but again, neither these burglaries nor the murder could be linked to Hogan.

Without hard forensic evidence to prove anything different, there seemed little more police could do to create a persuasive case for Hogan being a killer. Resources are finite in investigations like this; it wasn't an important or high-profile case. The reality is that the murder of an old man in his home soon drops off the media radar. The sheer volume of objects in Hogan's lock-up also presented a practical problem: it would be too expensive and time-consuming to send it all for forensic analysis. Without any new developments to inform the next stage of the process, the case had, as they say, gone cold.

The day after my initial meeting with Steve and Jo, I returned to the station and sat alone in a small room to take a look at the crime scene evidence collected at the time of Malcolm Johns' death. Looking at photographs of someone who has been killed – especially if their end was met in a particularly humiliating or brutal way – isn't something that feels any more normal the more you do it. It's like catching your neighbour in her nightie or walking in on someone you don't know when they're on the toilet. There's a deep, primal sense that here is something you were never supposed to see.

Death is such an intimate and private moment – arguably the most private of all. Sometimes I see not only the outside of victims' bodies but the insides too: organs that have spilled out, brains that have been smashed in, genitals that have been exposed or mutilated. There is surely nothing more intimate than a person's insides. The feeling of regret, that I – a stranger – have seen them like this, doesn't ever recede.

Crime scene pictures document in painstaking detail the place where something unspeakable has happened. Over half of all homicides take place in some sort of dwelling, so I'm often taking a tour of people's homes.

Once a crime has been discovered, forensic teams go in and carefully peel back the layers of the site, like the skin of an onion. At each layer, evidence is documented and meticulously labelled, stripping the whole thing back, taking investigators and others involved in the process further to the heart of the matter.

Sometimes a victim's actual heart is photographed, too, if the pictures also go on to document the post-mortem examination of the body. The pathologist slices the body down the front in one long incision and the organs are removed and photographed. Another incision is made at the back of the skull so that the brain can be examined, and at every stage there are photographs.

It is a dismal fact that some of the photographs I see are of babies or very young children. The Home Office Homicide Index consistently shows that children under one year old have the highest rate of victimization or death by homicide per million population. That means that a person is more likely to meet a violent death in the first 12 months of life than at any other age. Almost always they are killed by a parent or step-parent.

When I'm looking at a picture of a body, I like to have a brief conversation in my head with the person they once were. I say something like: Hello, I'm so sorry this happened to you. Now let's see what you can tell me, shall we? It sounds silly, but I do it to be polite, to feel that I have shown them respect, even though this person is dead and has no idea that I am silently conversing with their photograph. I do it as much for their relatives and families as for them, or maybe just for me. I don't have any religious or romantic notions about death, but still, humans should go out with someone holding their hand, not with violence. A body is someone's flesh and blood. So I suppose it's an attempt of sorts to keep a respectful bedside manner about me.

It takes a couple of seconds for my mind to register what I'm seeing. My body always registers it first, and it takes an unpleasant moment for the burst of electricity across my skin – the 'galvanic skin response', the body's instantaneous reaction to stress – to subside. I am looking at the end result of what has happened. I begin to attempt to reconstruct *how* it happened in my head, creating a timeline of likely thoughts, decisions and actions of the people involved. That said, I'm not trying to 'get into the mind' of anyone, like some mystical shaman – it's more like putting myself in their shoes. I'm trying to gain some practical knowledge that will guide me to ask the right questions or direct me to the next piece of evidence, and be of use in answering the questions I've been issued with. I am always aware that what I am seeing isn't all there is. And yet it is often all you have. A game of psychological join-the-dots when someone has rubbed out more than a few of the dots.

It never gets more normal, but the longer you look,

the more you can habituate, and see with a detached professional interest. Like any daunting task, you get through it by breaking it down into component parts rather than a whole, focusing on small aspects, taking it one step at a time. Concentrate on the details like this and eventually – if you're lucky – the full picture comes into view.

*

I carefully laid out all the images taken at Malcolm Johns' house. It was a two-bedroom terrace with a narrow staircase that took you up to the landing, delivering you directly outside the 'back bedroom' where Mr Johns had been sleeping. He had apparently suffered with sleep apnoea for years and snored loudly, often waking his wife – and himself – up in the night. So Mrs Johns had decamped to the bedroom at the front of the house. (She still wore earplugs every night, so that on the night he was killed she didn't hear a thing until the fire alarm went off. Then she ran in to find her husband dead on the floor.)

Pictures of his bed showed the orthopaedic pillow soaked in blood and the headboard covered in upward splatters. He'd been killed while still in bed, and his body then moved to the floor. His head was between the end right-hand corner of the bed and the foot of the mirrored wardrobes that ran the width of the room. His body was slightly rolled over, one arm out in front, shoulder hunched in an almost insouciant pose, the other underneath his torso, raising him up like a little pedestal. It was an unnatural position, as if he had been dropped quickly onto the floor and left there, the whole thing made stranger by the way it was reflected in the mirrored wardrobes. Twin corpses.

He'd taken at least four vicious blows to the back of his head with something heavy – the pictures showed how his skull had collapsed in on itself.

The length of his body was photographed in detail as is normal, but of particular interest were his hands. Two fingers on his right hand were distorted, smashed out of line, and on both hands the fingers bore deep bruising and blood where parts of the skin had burst open with what looked like the force of a blow from a heavy object. These were not the kinds of defensive wounds you expect to see if someone has raised their hands to protect themselves. The pathologists had confirmed it: his hands had been clasped behind his head when the blows had been struck.

Pictures also showed how part of the rug that he had ended up on and a patch on the leg of his pyjamas were singed. It looked like the killer had hastily tried to set fire to the fabric, in an attempt, no doubt, to destroy any trace of himself on the victim, but without any lighter fluid or accelerant it hadn't caught. It had caused the fire alarm to go off, though.

I could see no practical reason for moving Malcolm Johns' body from the bed. It was a cumbersome and unnecessary act. And when behaviour serves no practical purpose, it most likely serves a psychological need. Why was he dropped there, in front of the mirror?

The Scottish serial killer Dennis Nilsen was responsible for the deaths of at least 12 young men. He liked to engage in a pseudo relationship with the bodies of his victims – he liked to bathe his dead victims, dress them up and follow certain rituals involving their corpses. In his extensive and articulate confessions Nilsen talked about being bullied at school by a boy who later drowned. The young Nilsen recalled feeling both jubilant and aroused as he watched the boy's semi-naked body being carried onto shore. This boy, who had once inspired fear in Nilsen, was no longer able to assert himself, reduced to passively receiving the attentions of a nurse and a mortician. This defining moment inspired in him a lifelong fascination with a painting called *The Raft of the Medusa*, which became the inspiration for his increasingly deviant sexual fantasies. The 1819 painting by Théodore Géricault depicts the aftermath of the wreckage of the French naval frigate *Medusa*, and shows an old man on a makeshift raft holding the naked, pale body of a dead young man.

I once had a disconcertingly casual conversation with Dennis Nilsen while he was serving his life sentence at HMP Full Sutton. In his soft Scottish burr, he told me that strangling or drowning his victims was a means not an end.

The most rewarding element of his grotesque rituals was picking up his victims and standing in front of a mirror with them cradled in his arms so he could see himself holding them. He said he liked to see their bodies in a similar pose to that of the bully who he'd watched being pulled out of the water – limp, unresisting. And himself, supreme. Staring at his reflection in the mirror as he held his victims, their arms flopping down at their sides, he took a mental picture – a visual trophy of sorts – which he could call upon when he felt inadequate and wanted to return to this powerful moment in his mind.

Had the killer gone to the trouble of pulling Malcolm Johns out of bed so he could see himself holding the body in front of the mirror? Did he crave the same visual confirmation of his own power over another human being that Nilsen had?

*

My next step was to watch the interviews with Hogan that police had conducted after he'd been arrested for the storage unit robbery. I had the accompanying transcript in my hands, but so much useful behavioural information is not recorded on paper, so I put it down and just watched the video.

Steve was right. Hogan had given little away in those interviews. The grainy split-screen footage showed him sitting with his legs crossed and his hands grasping his knee, an unconscious way of making sure his body didn't leak any incriminating information. He was a jar with the lid screwed on tight.

It was an almost textbook example of PEACE, as the interview process used by the police is known. The letters stand for Preparation/planning; Explaining the purpose of the interview; Asking for the suspect's account of the evidence/what happened; Challenging their account/concluding; Evaluation. It's a framework officers use to ensure that as much useful information as possible is gathered in the interview process. Every operational officer in the country gets PEACE training, and in recent years the technique has developed into several tiers of training, tailored specifically to certain areas of crime.

I watched Hogan as he answered the questions. He took two long, slow breaths before he said anything. It reminded me of what I had been trained to do as an expert witness in court – what we call the 'courtroom swivel'. When a barrister asks me a question, I don't react straight away. I take a few seconds as I turn to look at the jury or the judge before I give my answer. Not only is it correct protocol to address the judge and jury, not the lawyer, it slows the whole process down. I don't turn back to the barrister until I've finished saying what I want to say. I can't be drawn into a careless, quick-fire exchange if I take the vital time I need to ensure my response is on point and conveys what I want it to.

Being questioned under pressure, and with such a lot riding on your answers, is a taxing situation for anyone to find themselves in, so it makes sense that you carve out those extra seconds to collect your thoughts.

> **Police officer:** Can you explain to us how you come to be in possession of Malcolm Johns' watch?
> **Hogan:** [*breathe one, two*] I don't recall exactly, I buy lots of things from lots of people. It was probably part of a job lot. I don't recall having seen it. [*blink*]

After a couple of hours, Hogan's non-committal and carefully constructed answers started taking their toll on the interviewing officers. I could see them getting weary and their body language becoming more confrontational – as were the questions. Studies repeatedly show that even the most highly trained police interviewers can lapse into interrupting the suspect, asking closed questions or demanding answers that confirm their assumptions about what happened.

The first officer pushed a photograph of Mr Johns' body across the table towards Hogan and then sat back in his chair and folded his arms. The muscles in Hogan's jaw tensed slightly.

> **Police officer:** You killed him, didn't you?
> **Hogan:** [*breathe one, two*] …not me.

Police officer: You battered Malcolm Johns to death in his bed.

Hogan: *[breathe one, two]* …not me, I didn't batter anyone.

I noticed Hogan make gentle, affirmative nods to each question before readjusting his position, hunched over and folding his arms in mirror image to his accuser. This was a brief but telling contradiction between his verbal denial and the language of his body. But neither officer saw it – one was looking at the photograph and the other was watching her colleague.

*

Six weeks later, I was at the station again for the second round of questioning. Hogan had been transferred out of his category C (resettlement) prison for a two-day trip to the custody suite at the police station. I caught a brief glimpse of him as he was booked into his new accommodation by the custody officer. He seemed smaller than the person I'd watched on the video, shrunken and more gaunt than he'd been in those first interviews.

In the meantime, Steve and I had devised a detailed interview plan. I had suggested that since Hogan had dug his heels in so visibly (what psychologists call 'psychological reactance') when he had been pushed by officers in his original interviews to admit guilt (and let's not forget, he could still be innocent – the point of an interview is to elicit reliable information, not necessarily extract a confession), letting him take the reins in this interview would produce better results. The storage unit robbery had shown us that he was a man who liked to be in control, so we decided to give him just that and see if it got him talking. That meant leaving longer silences and waiting for him to speak, using only the minimum of prompts if necessary, even asking Hogan what he felt would help the police to talk about, and generally appearing to be more submissive.

All interviews, whether of victims or suspects, are governed by the Police and Criminal Evidence Act (PACE). This is the legislative framework that ensures everyone coming into contact with the investigative process is treated humanely and fairly. To avoid any suggestion that admissions made during interrogation were extracted under pressure, it requires police to make audio and visual recordings of interviews for use as evidence, and it allows certain experts and professionals, like me, to watch proceedings without being in the room. It was the first time I'd been in a custody suite since acting as an appropriate adult (someone who sits in on police station interviews with vulnerable suspects) as a student, and I recognized the atmosphere, alive with pure, steely focus from everyone.

I took my seat alongside Steve and a typist in a small interview room and watched on the video screen as a detective superintendent and another officer settled down across the table from Hogan and his solicitor. They began going through the usual formalities 'for the tape'. Hogan took up position – as I had seen him do previously – with his hands clasped together over his knees, rigid.

It took an hour or so, but when given the opportunity to lead the way, Hogan began to relax into the process and talk spontaneously, particularly about how he had been wrongly convicted of the storage facility incident. He kept asserting that the police should be talking to some of his drinking acquaintances about that matter and a number of potentially valuable items that had been found in his lock-up. He was especially irritated about his collection of antique weapons, which, he said, had been unfairly destroyed when he was sentenced.

He seemed keen to make his indignation known. The interviewers stuck to the strategy and, with no prompting, Hogan repeatedly returned to complaining about how these possessions, including the imitation firearm believed to have been the one used in the robbery, had been seized. He kept returning to the fact that they had been destroyed. 'I can't believe they destroyed them. They weren't illegal, were they? They were destroyed, weren't they?'

He wanted confirmation that these weapons had gone. This was interesting – why was it still so important to him now, more than four years after his arrest? Without being pushed, he had willingly led us to something that clearly mattered to him.

The interview spread over two days. Hogan was allowed to ramble in detail and at length about what was important to him. When it came to more direct matters, he continued to give closed responses and brief, indirect denials. Occasionally his response seemed scripted, as if he had rehearsed the answers to these questions already. They were, after all, easily anticipated: 'Me kill Malcolm Johns? I wouldn't hit an old man, I'm not the sort to hurt a fly.'

But Hogan hadn't been expecting the last question the detective asked him, delivered almost as an afterthought as he was preparing to finish up. We had agreed beforehand that he would ask it in just this way, the so-called 'silver bullet' to catch Hogan unawares.

'Did you pick Mr Johns up and look at yourself in the mirror when you were holding him?'

I paid close attention as Hogan's mouth stretched sideways, a fleeting expression of fear. His head bobbed as his whole body shifted. He pushed his chair back against the wall as if to physically distance himself from the question. Suddenly he was flustered. 'What are you trying to say?' he spat. Then, sucking air into his nostrils and closing his eyes, his voice dropped as he insisted: 'Not me, not me.' But his body had already contradicted his denial.

When someone is lying, especially if the truth might land them in prison, their brain is working overtime to make sure that whatever comes out of their mouth is bulletproof. Ask a high-stakes liar a question, and they'll need to make sure that what they say and do has the ring of absolute truth to it. But while their mind is conjuring up a plausible display, their body tends to instantaneously and unconsciously leak the truth. Sometimes even when they, like Hogan, are self-aware enough to take the time they need to reflect and choose a response.

In the 1960s, US lie detection expert Dr Paul Ekman first conducted analyses on physical reactions like those Hogan could not control in that moment. Behavioural analysts at the UK Emotional Intelligence Academy have since identified the 3-2-7 rule: if a suspect has a cluster of three reactions (for example, nodding, flushing and voice dropping in pitch), across two or more of the six channels that communicate emotional information (interactional style, voice, verbal content, facial expression, body movements and physiological changes) within seven seconds of the question, it is a reliable indication of deception. We didn't know about that then, only that Hogan's words had told us something his body wasn't agreeing with.

Hogan composed himself after a few moments, more deep breaths, and the interview was concluded. But his unusual reaction to that question, together with his eagerness to garner reassurance that his weapons had been destroyed, was enough for Steve and the team to feel that taking another look at the imitation firearm from the storage unit robbery would be a useful allocation of resources.

What they discovered was a game-changer. The replica had been forensically examined at the time of its discovery, and nothing of interest was found on it. In a rare display of efficiency, it had indeed been destroyed as ordered by the court. But as luck would have it, a large laundry bag belonging to Hogan that he had told us that his weapons had been wrapped in was still packaged up in storage along with some other unexamined possessions from the lock-up. The bag was analysed by forensics, who discovered the smallest amount of blood at the bottom of the lining – blood belonging to Malcolm Johns.

Hogan had battered Malcolm Johns to death, possibly with the butt of his replica pistol, and a tiny speck of blood from the attack had been sitting in the bottom of the bag ever since. With that key bit of evidence the team was able to pursue the case to prosecution, getting a conviction that would ensure that Hogan remained in prison for many years.

Answering Steve's call that day became the first small step on a new path for me. It would lead to a new strand of consultancy work, forging relationships with a number of police forces that would become a small but rewarding part of my private practice.

I will never know what triggered Hogan to kill Malcolm Johns. I suspect Johns challenged him in some way, said something to undermine Hogan's belief in himself as effective in controlling others, powerful enough to intrude upon them and take what he wanted. I do know that Hogan continued to protest his innocence, right up until the first day of his trial for Malcolm Johns' murder, changing his plea to 'guilty' at the last minute, holding on to the last bit of control he had.

CHAPTER 7
INSULTS AND INJURIES

The human brain is unprepossessing to look at – a pinky-grey wrinkled lump with the consistency of congealed porridge – but appearances are, of course, deceptive.
Professor Peter Kinderman, *The New Laws of Psychology*

Gary had a Sainsbury's bag for life that he carried with him wherever he went. It was bright orange plastic with a cartoon drawing of an elephant on it and a strapline that said 'I'm Strong and Sturdy'. Sometimes he had things in it, but he was in prison so the shopping wasn't great, and very often the bag was empty. It didn't matter to Gary. It was a bag for life and that meant it was his, for life.

I learned some time later that his mum would quietly replace his bag for life with a fresh one whenever the old one wore out or, as sometimes happened, other inmates stole or damaged it. He once smashed up his own cell after an inmate burned holes in the bag with a cigarette.

I had been asked by Gary's solicitor to review him; his family needed advice about how to help him move more effectively through the prison system, which seemed to them like a complex maze with no exits. Although he wasn't a lifer he might as well have been one, because Gary was serving an imprisonment for public protection (IPP) sentence – a jail term with no fixed end date.

These now-defunct sentences were introduced by former Home Secretary David Blunkett, presumably on an especially act-first-think-second day. They were intended to protect the public from offenders whose crimes were serious but didn't warrant a life sentence, and were applicable to 153 crimes, from affray to manslaughter. IPP sentences – abolished in 2012 yet many are still being served today – consisted of a minimum punitive term (known as a 'tariff') which offenders had to spend in prison, and bolted onto this was a further 99-year licence, meaning they could technically stay in prison for an extra 99 years – after the tariff has expired, they have to apply to and satisfy a parole board that they are fit for release.

Some ideas are best left on paper. The IPP model was applied far more widely than intended, and used in the wrong way by many courts. Swathes of offenders received short tariffs but went on to spend many extra years in prison, effectively being punished for crimes that they *might* commit, because they couldn't meet the demands of the parole board.

A three-person panel led by a judge, the parole board decides who can and cannot go home based on whether or not they are judged to pose a continuing risk to the public. But as the prison psychologist Robert A. Forde points out in his book *Bad Psychology*, we can predict statistically whether a person is likely to reoffend seriously with only around 70 per cent accuracy. This leaves an alarming void that the system likes to fill by prescribing offending behaviour courses, and assessing prisoners by their abilities to complete them and to wax lyrical about their reformed character during an interview.

I'd worked with Gary's solicitor, James, before – he was one of the good guys. It was 2009, I had a well-established private practice by then. I had cemented a reputation for myself among solicitors on the northern circuit for writing no-nonsense, jargon-free reports. I was particularly well known for providing straight-talking insight on cases involving serious or sexual violence or anything else in the realm of the psychologically obscure. James once called to instruct me in the case of a man who had been, among other things, dressing up a donkey in women's clothes stolen from his neighbour's washing line. 'I thought it sounded right up your street,' he'd said, with no apparent irony.

This was before austerity, when Legal Aid was available for those who needed it, and if a solicitor was concerned about the mental state of their client they'd ask you to prepare an independent report. Solicitors don't have an easy task. They have no specialist training in the area, yet it often falls to them to flag up if someone has mental health issues. Or indeed any issues. A solicitor involved in a case such as Gary's can find themselves being an agony aunt and confidante one minute and a surrogate parent and legal expert the next. I've known solicitors hold their clients' hands during paternity tests, and deliver hot coffee to their clients on the street in the morning so they turn up at court on time and vaguely sober. One solicitor I knew swapped clothes with a man who had a job interview, his first in a very long time. You quickly learn to recognize the ones who are doing the job well; in many ways they become your colleagues.

Although they always want the best outcome for their clients, whereas I am entirely independent, a good solicitor acknowledges and appreciates my non-partisan opinion. I had good professional relationships with a number of law practices across the north, but James – a beefy man without a hair on his head, whose entire scalp rippled when he smiled – always stood out as someone who gave his clients both realism and respect.

James explained that Gary was unlikely to ever be judged as fit for release by a parole board due to impulsive behaviour that was getting him into regular scrapes with other prisoners. He'd stolen inmates' food from their trays at meal times; sometimes he ate it and other times threw it across the landing – risky when your fellow diners like to enforce mealtime etiquette by punching you in the face. He had recently been in trouble for mooning, pulling his trousers down and showing his bare behind to anyone unfortunate enough to see it during wing association time (when all the inmates get to socialize).

Gary's popularity with the other prisoners was further reduced by what seemed to be the literal way he interpreted situations. Not only did he take his bag for life at its word, but when other inmates asked him what he was in prison for, he would tell them – a truth that was never well received.

Gary was what's known inside as a 'nonce'. He had sexually assaulted a 13-year-old girl, by touching her while on a bus. In the spurious hierarchy of prison honour, Gary was considered the worst kind of low-life there is (top of the pile are armed robbers – robbing a bank is considered to be a noble, Robin Hood-style redistribution of wealth). A wiser sex-offender would have kept their crime to themselves, or come up with a more crowd-pleasing cover story. But it seemed like Gary couldn't do that – he was compelled to answer with the facts. Facts that, more often than not, were met with a verbal or physical attack.

Gary was perpetually getting into fights with fellow inmates. I saw him twice with black eyes, and had a number of meetings cancelled at the last minute because he was 'down the block': in the segregated cells where inmates are sent as punishment. Loss of privileges and confinement is the default response to violation of the rules in prison, and for Gary it often meant being locked in a block cell for the majority of the day. In a block cell you are permitted to keep a book, if you own one, a prison issue toothbrush, plastic mug, plate, bowl and plastic cutlery. You have a towel, some toothpaste and half a bar of prison soap. There is no radio, no visitors, very little interaction with other inmates or staff and definitely no bag for life.

To add to Gary's problems, he hadn't managed to complete any of the offending-behaviour programmes that the parole board expected him to. This was his second prison and the first hadn't run any of the programmes specified in his sentence plan. He had been given a set of imaginary hoops to jump through – a familiar predicament for many IPP prisoners. At his current prison he had spent nearly a year on a waiting list to take part in the Enhanced Thinking Skills programme, a group that teaches problem-solving and reasoning skills, but had only managed to complete two sessions of it; he had urinated on the floor in the second session and then refused to get out of his cell for the rest. Not only had Gary failed quite spectacularly in being taught how to think by his offending behaviour programme, he hadn't managed to attend any education or work programmes with any consistency either. So what had originally been a ten-month sentence had turned into nearly four years.

James, and Gary's family, wanted to know how they could help Gary turn a corner, one with at least a glimpse of an eventual release on the horizon.

*

My heart sank just thinking about it. Square-peg prisoners and the penal system don't tend to find happy endings. I could make all kinds of suggestions in order to facilitate Gary's more satisfactory behaviour, but in the end it would boil down to available resources – and they are critically thin on the ground in the majority of prisons. Gary was never going to be the model prisoner or develop the level of eloquence needed to endear himself to parole board assessors. But I hoped that I could at least provide some objective information about his level of dangerousness, and what sort of package might be needed to keep him out of trouble if released, which might then inform a discussion when his case was next up for review.

James sent me the witness statements that were taken from the people involved in the incident on the bus. Depositions like this are difficult documents to make sense of at first. Police interviews are transcribed verbatim, without any punctuation; sheets of A4 with endless speech typed all in capital letters. It looks like an angry missive from an old relative who has just learned to use email. The unstructured layout somehow makes the facts of the story harder to find, hidden within an upper-case forest.

What came across immediately was the utter mayhem that had unfolded on the bus that evening. It was 7pm and a group of four young teens – ages ranging from 12 to 15 – had been to the cinema (they'd seen a *Pirates of the Caribbean* film, prophetic, because it sounded like a kind of mutiny had unfolded) and were travelling home. They'd got bags of Haribo and cans of fizzy drink and were all sitting upstairs, dispersed across different seats, the way teenagers seem to do.

The children's statements described how Gary was also upstairs, was asleep and had an orange carrier bag on his lap. I gathered from their insensitive descriptions of him that, aside from his unconventional choice of sleeping arrangements, Gary also looked unusual. One of the girls had dared another of them to touch him on the face – a dare which had set in motion the series of events which would lead to Gary's incarceration.

Another girl's statement said:

RACHEL TOUCHED HIM ON THE FACE AND HE WOKE UP AND THEN DARREN SHOUTED FRAGGLE AT HIM AND THEN HE SAID TO RACHEL DO YOU FANCY ME OR SOMETHING? AND THEN WE WERE ALL RUNNING AWAY SAYING GET LOST YOU WEIRDO AND RACHEL STARTED SCREAMING AND HE GRABBED HER AND

PUT HIS HAND UP HER SKIRT AND WAS SQUEEZING HER THERE AND THEN CARL RAN PAST HIM AND HE TOUCHED CARL'S BUM BUT CARL WAS JUST LAUGHING.

All the statements described the same moment: how Gary had woken from his sleep and began to clamber over seats, grabbing chaotically at the children, in particular the girl called Rachel, who described how he cornered her before forcefully pinching her between her legs through her underwear. Seeing this more sinister turn in events, another passenger had pinned Gary into the nearest seat long enough for the bus to stop and the driver to call the police.

Gary fitted the dirty old man on the bus stereotype, albeit one in his 30s. The oddball stranger we warn our children about, who women hope to protect themselves from by walking with their keys placed between their fingers, Wolverine-style. The latest Crime Survey for England and Wales (CSEW) found that around 20 per cent of women and 4 per cent of men taking part reported being sexually assaulted in some way since the age of 16, estimating around 650,000 assaults in 2017 on this group of victims alone. Logic dictates that there must be a roughly equivalent number of perpetrators.

They can't all be peculiar characters on the back of a bus or dark figures in an alleyway. The idea of a sexual assault taking place at the hands of a stranger, and involving extreme violence or the threat of weapons, is, for the most part at least, a myth. The even less palatable truth is that in the majority of sexual assault and rape cases, whether adults or children are the target, the perpetrators are people who the victim knows: family members, partners, work colleagues or acquaintances. Sexual harassment – verbal abuse such as cat-calling and other forms of bullying – is rife in public spaces, but hands-on sexual crimes are most likely to take place in the victim's own home.

With the children's statements fresh in my mind I went to meet Gary in the prison where he was being held (a two-hour drive from his parents' home in Bolton). I had arranged to meet with him on the prison's VPU (vulnerable prisoner unit). Gary was 'on the numbers', what used to be known as Rule 43 but is now Prison Rule 45: Removal from Association. Inmates are separated when it is deemed necessary for their own protection. Sex offenders are often VPs, as are police informers, former police officers and those with large drug debts, but they are also often prisoners with learning disabilities or other discernible differences that might make them easy targets for predators. VPs are usually housed in a dedicated unit away from the main wing, or unlocked from their cells at different times of day from the other prisoners.

I sat in the small, bare meeting room waiting for him,

a square Perspex window making sure my time with Gary would be observable throughout by the guard who stood like a sentinel in the corridor. Seeing me temporarily unoccupied, the guard came in for a chat, the allure of a new face presumably being just too much to resist. Leaning casually against the wall, he explained that the demand for the VPU at this prison far exceeded the available space so they didn't like to keep Gary there for long. But whenever he returned to the main wing, it would be a matter of days before he would have another bout of verbal incontinence, revealing his offence details to anyone who asked, and he'd find himself back to the VPU or the punishment cells. The guard told me this and rolled his eyes as if to say how incredibly stupid Gary was for telling the truth; the bittersweet contradiction of a prisoner being so honest it got him into trouble was obviously lost on him.

When Gary eventually came in it was very slowly; he was a heavy mass, doughy and soft, and he lurched towards me with his arms out in front of him, like an elderly person who had lost their walking frame. I noticed his bag for life, scraggy and faded, folded in his left hand, together with a letter from James reminding him of my visit. I put my right hand out to shake his, but he surprised me by patting me on the head instead, ruffling my hair with his fingers as if I was a Labrador. He was tall – at least six foot – and at five foot three I was considerably shorter than him. In this job you get used to your personal space being invaded and to social conventions and politeness being on rations. By that stage in my career there were very few insults that hadn't been thrown my way. So I didn't say anything and held my hand out again, but once more he patted me on the head. So I took a step backwards and said breezily: 'You can stop that now, please, Gary.' He put his hand down by his side, as if I'd slapped the back of his hand. I felt conflicted. Being petted like a dog would usually be a guaranteed hackle-raiser for me, but I didn't feel that he was being disrespectful or trying to intimidate me.

I asked him to sit down – gesturing him to the usual uninviting plastic chair, wondering privately if it would hold under Gary's considerable load. We went through the cursory introductions. I noticed his speech was quite poorly articulated, with noticeable derhotacization, meaning he had difficulty pronouncing 'r' sounds. He was Gawee, not Gary.

I asked him how he was and rather unexpectedly he launched into a diatribe about his legs. He was very concerned about them, they felt weak and wobbly. As he talked I wrote notes, and whenever I put my pen down he picked it up and started to doodle the same thing repeatedly, his full name and an outline rendering of a stripy cat. I had to keep asking for my pen back and wait for him to finish his masterpiece before returning it. He didn't seem to remember not to do it. This is 'utilization behaviour', where someone uses the appropriate behaviour associated with an object, but at an inappropriate time. He was only doing what everybody does with a pen, but his timing and understanding of the context was off.

As with any job, in psychology part of being effective is knowing where your skillset ends and someone else's is required. I'm not a neuropsychologist – someone who understands brain health and the way it impacts behaviour – but I began to wonder if perhaps Gary's problems were more physical than purely psychological.

I had asked to see his medical records, but the prison had nothing on file. When he had arrived at reception in his first prison, Gary hadn't been able to tell them which GP he was registered with, and it looked as though the matter had been left at that. No one knew his medical history, so anything that had happened before prison had essentially been forgotten. (This isn't an unusual scenario by any means – it's not how it should be, but it is how it is. Our creaking, overburdened public services don't always succeed at the fabled joined-up thinking.) He'd gone through the standard quick screen for mental health issues – nine questions in all – on three occasions and he hadn't reported anything significant on each. There were a few notes from visits to the prison GP but they were in connection to his vague complaints about his legs and minor injuries. I noticed he'd had cigarette burns on his legs and severe bruising on his back – things that had been done to him by other prisoners.

I knew I needed to get a clearer picture of his background if I was going to understand what was driving Gary's disinhibited behaviour. But the in-depth clinical interview with him that I wanted wasn't coming easily. I couldn't get any meaningful information from him. He just kept talking about his legs, and the fact that his cell door didn't have a handle on the inside, just a metal plate where a handle ought to be. When I probed for details about his life before prison he'd say, 'Mum knows. Ask Mum.' He deferred to her almost every time I asked him anything: 'Have you ever had a job, Gary?' or 'Which school did you go to?' He would repeat, 'Mum knows.' It was clear he had relied heavily on her, even as an adult. I needed to meet his mum.

*

Having an independent practice allowed me to make that sort of call. I had achieved a freedom of my own; I was mistress of my own schedule and could keep the hours I wanted to – useful for me at that stage as I could work around a Ménière's attack if I had one. Useful for my clients, too, because I could provide the sort of individualized service I wanted to give them, and do things like get in the car and visit someone's mum. As an employee there had rarely been the time, the money nor the outside-the-box mindset that allows for the sort of investigative approach I felt was needed in Gary's case.

The flip side, of course, is that as a private practitioner you have less time to build therapeutic relationships with clients. You helicopter in at your moment, conduct your interviews, make your recommendations, and often you are out again just as quickly. You have the satisfaction of a job done thoroughly but it can feel isolated, you miss out on the longer-term connections and day-to-day interaction, not only with your workmates, but also with your patients and clients.

So the following week I found myself pulling up outside Gary's mum's house in Bolton. I've been inside plenty of people's houses with my work and met many a concerned and caring parent, but it's hard to remember a more homely visit. Standing at the front door, the brass knocker beyond shiny, I saw Ann pull the net curtains in the window to one side to check it was me. She opened the door but kept it on the chain and said: 'Is that you Kerry, love?' – like I was a long-lost daughter she couldn't quite believe had returned at last. I held up my ID card through the gap but she was opening the door by then.

Inside, she had a wall plaque that read: 'This home is clean enough to be healthy and dirty enough to be happy'. My grandmother had the same one on her kitchen wall and for a moment I was transported back to her house. Even though I'd never been there before I was immediately full of nostalgia in Ann's home.

She'd gone full hostess with the nest of tables fanned out in a decadent flourish and a pot of tea and a plate of custard creams all waiting for me, the whole tableau unfathomably swathed in layers of kitchen roll. We sat down and the pain poured out of her like tea from the pot: she had obviously been needing to talk to someone for a long time. She didn't understand the IPP sentence and why Gary was still in prison four years later. He wasn't a sex offender; how could they call him that? Tears sprang from her pale green eyes as she asked me this. She obviously found that particular reality very difficult to deal with.

It's easy to forget that offenders' families experience their own kind of trauma when their loved ones go to prison. Feelings of bereavement and isolation, shame and guilt, are all part of the unhappy mix. Matters were made worse for Gary's mum as he was being held in a prison so far away from her. Gary's dad had died, and she didn't drive, so she barely saw her son at all.

One year, she told me, close to Christmas, she'd made the journey to see Gary with some presents for him. When she got there he was in segregation, so she couldn't see him. She tried to leave the gifts for him. Handing them back to her a prison officer had said: 'Sorry, he's been a naughty boy.'

I asked her about Gary's past and his medical history

and she told me that he had been 'very poorly with cancer' as a child. Here was something, at last. But it was clear she didn't have an in-depth understanding of his problems or what they might have meant for him as an adult. She just wanted me to know that she had done everything right. She talked about looking after him and caring for him when he had chemotherapy as a boy. I got the feeling she'd been well-meaning but also possibly smothering, so determined to look after her child that no one else was allowed to. She got a box of photographs out and showed me pictures of him as a child, in the garden with his grandad, his school portraits in the generic brown cardboard frame that I recognized from my own school pictures. Gary had got his five GCSEs. She had given him as normal and respectable a childhood as she could, and she really needed me to understand that.

Although she couldn't tell me much more she was able to point me in the direction of the family GP practice, and I was then able to begin gathering together the full details of his medical history. It's not an aspect of my job that requires any psychological insight or judgement, but hunting down paperwork – medical files, police records, witness statements from previous offences, care records, school reports and educational assessments – is a significant part of doing it well. Back then this was especially true, because as a private practitioner I had only my own resources to rely on and couldn't easily access patient files. It's a surprisingly time-consuming and mentally draining task, often dealing with desk staff who consider sharing any kind of information a personal failure, and who are working under strict regulatory guidelines about patient confidentiality. Emails must be sent and confirmations received and permissions granted, not just from the person concerned but often from multiple people, some of whom no longer work where you want them to work or who are too busy and stressed to spare time for a stranger, especially one who is asking about someone they haven't seen or thought about for 20 years.

It took me nearly two months to finally have the medical files I needed in my hands. The collection of papers and documents I eventually sat down one evening to digest was 14 inches thick. I made notes on his records late into the night, Gary's story coming into focus so sharply and urgently that I called James first thing the next morning.

*

At four years old Gary had been diagnosed with acute lymphoblastic leukaemia, and had received chemotherapy until he was seven. He'd also had an intensive course of cranial radiotherapy – a treatment commonly given to people with his particular kind of leukaemia, as they are at a higher risk of it affecting the brain.

I'm no neuroscientist but I did some topline research that evening and learned that a potential complication of cranial radiotherapy is damage to the frontal lobe area of the brain, the part that sits just behind your eyes, which can impact and impair almost all aspects of executive functioning – the mental skills that help humans with everything from memory and flexible thinking (making judgements, learning cause and effect) to controlling urges and impulses.

Gary had presumably sustained damage to this 'control panel' area of his brain as a consequence of his cancer treatment, but it hadn't been detected for years. He attended mainstream schools, but missed a lot due to hospital treatment and struggled to make any friends (a particularly pitiful note from his school nurse described how he'd once been thrown into a wheelie bin by his classmates). He struggled generally to keep up and left school at 16 with five GCSEs, all at the lowest pass grades. I noted he'd been assessed by a child psychologist, when he was ten years old, who gave him an IQ score of around 85: low average. By the time he was assessed again by a neuropsychologist at 25, his IQ had dropped to 72. Something progressive was clearly happening to Gary.

At one stage he was admitted to psychiatric services following an episode where he'd been found wandering the streets, disoriented and confused. The police had picked him up. He was described as both 'apathetic' and 'hyperactive' but 'there are no indicators of mental illness...this young man has behavioural disturbance'. More time in mental health services passed until eventually, aged 29, Gary was sent to his local brain injuries rehabilitation services for assessment. Years before the incident on the bus and Gary's conviction, he was formally diagnosed with frontal lobe syndrome. Tap this into Google and you learn that symptoms can include over-exuberant, childish conduct and inappropriate sexual behaviour. Sufferers can also lack the ability to switch ideas easily, typically becoming attached to words or gestures long after they have ceased to be socially relevant or appropriate. In addition, a meningioma tumour was growing in the lining of his brain compressing his frontal lobe, exacerbating the changes and deterioration in his behaviour.

Meningioma tumours are generally benign but the bigger they get, the more problems they cause, so doctors told Gary that they wanted to remove this tumour with surgery as soon as possible. I noted there were concerns about the safety of the procedure due to his weight – compulsive eating is also a symptom of frontal lobe syndrome – and that he suffered with sleep apnoea. However, there was no doubt that Gary needed surgery to remove this growth.

At that point Gary's notes came to an end, becoming a series of copies of letters sent to him detailing dates and times of appointments. There were seven or eight saying the same thing: 'You failed to attend your appointment, please contact us so we can reschedule.' It was clear he had never had the surgery.

It seems an obvious point, but the simple inclusion of relatives and families in the custody process can provide such useful information about the behaviour and condition of an inmate. The proportion of people with brain injuries estimated to be in the prison system at the moment is between 10 and 20 per cent. It's thought that around 30 per cent of all UK prisoners have a learning disability or an autistic spectrum disorder. People aged 60 or over are the fastest-growing age group in the British prison estate, and these prisoners are much more likely to be affected by neurological conditions like dementia and Parkinson's. British prisons – with the exception of a very small number of progressive institutions – don't know what to do with them, if they identify the problem correctly in the first place. Not only are those with these misunderstood conditions more likely to find themselves caught up in the criminal justice system, but, once banged up, they can find themselves in a Catch-22 situation; the prison environment makes it almost impossible for them to achieve the squeaky-clean behaviour expected of them. This is especially true for people on the autistic spectrum, for whom the cacophony of light and sound that is prison can be genuine torment. But their families know their stories. A little involvement of relatives could transform the prison experience for everyone involved.

Sometimes you show up to do a job and you realize that what needs doing is something completely different. Gary didn't need to see a psychologist, he needed to see a neurosurgeon as a matter of urgency, and James contacted the prison to let them know what had, or rather what hadn't, happened. My assessment was put on hold while medics got to grips with Gary's physical problems. I would meet him again post-op and we would continue to work on a risk assessment and possible pathway for his release.

Two months later I got a call from his mum. Gary had been transferred out of the prison to have surgery, but he had had a stroke while recovering from the operation, and died three weeks later.

*

The forensic psychologist in private practice shuttles in and out of people's lives and stories. I hear of former patients dying from time to time; often it's suicide, a drugs overdose or just general poor health. I don't spend enough time with most of my clients to form significant relationships. I'll often hear myself saying to them, at the end of a piece of work: 'In the best possible way, I hope we never meet again.' And it's often the case that we don't. It's the prison and hospital staff, those who work more closely with inmates and patients, who share more meaningful connections. And yet there is always a pause for reflection when a former patient dies.

I had a clutch of photographs Gary's mum had given me – the pictures of him as a child that she'd insisted I take with me last time I'd seen her – and I wanted to return them in person rather than send them. Nothing goes against the natural order of things more than the loss of a child, and I felt this woman had reached out to me with a degree of trust when I had visited her. Taking the pictures back felt like the right thing to do.

The best china was out again when I dropped by. There was a sense that a burden had been lifted. She was chatty, and keen to tell me the story of what had happened since I'd last seen her: it seemed that Gary hadn't ever told her about the need for surgery. He had obviously been scared, she said, and threw away the letters until eventually they stopped coming. He hadn't been to the doctor's for three years before the incident on the bus, so he was obviously not well. What had happened that day was a 'brain cough', as she called it. He was poorly and that was why he had done what he did.

She had constructed a version of events that made everything feel better for her and, although a part of me wanted to, I wasn't going to pick holes in it at this stage. I accepted that she had found a way to be at peace with what Gary had done. While his brain damage explained his failure to think through the consequences of his behaviour – the hardware causing blips in the programmes it implements – I believe there were other things he could have done, many ideas that he might have acted upon that day, that didn't involve sexually assaulting a child.

Reductionism, the idea that our behaviour is determined by nothing more than the biochemical processes of our brains, enjoys a certain amount of popularity in some scientific circles. It's a compelling notion – that there is ultimately no such thing as free will. That the determined nature of behaviour is just more obvious in those like Gary. For Ann, the explanation that 'his brain made him do it' was a salve for her grief. And her shame. Ignoring all of the complexities of human experience and environmental influence that combine to create a person's thoughts and actions was a clean and efficient way to wipe off the stain on his name that she found so distressing. I wish they did, but the cut-and-dry explanations that the families of offenders want to hear rarely exist.

As I was finishing my biscuit she asked me if I'd like to see Gary's ashes. I didn't especially, if I was honest – but before I had a chance to answer, she'd reached down the side of the sofa and pulled out a carrier bag, the brass urn holding Gary peeking out of the top of it. I wasn't quite sure what to say and I almost patted it, like Gary had patted me. Then I noticed the bag – it was bright orange, with a picture of an elephant on it that looked very familiar. Gary's final resting place was in his Sainsbury's bag for life. 'It's what he would have wanted,' she said. And she was absolutely right.

CHAPTER 8
A MAN'S WORLD

Men are afraid that women will laugh at them.
Women are afraid that men will kill them.
Margaret Atwood

I have clear-cut evidence that Kerry Daynes is a liar. I know for a fact that she is capable of lying. At worst it brings into question her credentials as an Expert Witness.

A biography about Kerry Daynes...Have you ever been conned by an expert? Has your life ever been destroyed by a so-called 'expert' or have your family and friends been destroyed by such people?

She is not the sharpest tool in the box but what the hell, she is a redhead, attractive and she has big tits. So what if her bum does look big in certain clothes.

More to follow...stay tuned.

I put my mug down and read the words on the screen in front of me again, the feeling that this was something quite ugly creeping through me. Lies written about me by someone I had never met, on a website that appeared to be in my name. What the hell was this?

A week earlier I'd received a Facebook message request from someone I didn't recognize. It was 2011 and Facebook was still quite new to me. I got, and still get, a lot of friend and message requests from people I don't know and normally I pay them little attention. It was a dreary Saturday morning in September, I was still in wake-up mode and my mind was a bit fuzzy around the edges, even though I was on my second cup of Yorkshire tea.

It said: 'I am not sure how you will take this but I have started a website for you.' Right. I usually appreciate a bold elevator pitch but not this one – I was suddenly very much awake. It was true I didn't have a website of my own, but I hadn't yet felt I needed one.

My private practice had been steadily growing for almost ten years by then. It was four years after I had met Gary and there had been many more prison visits. I had a healthy portfolio of consultancy and training work, as well as private clients and my work with the courts as an expert witness. I'd built a strong reputation for myself as a direct and honest psychologist, and as a result had also begun to make appearances on crime documentaries and series as a talking head. This TV work had come along unexpectedly in 2005 when I'd been asked by a news programme to comment on the case of teenager Brian Blackwell, who had been convicted of the manslaughter of his parents. I had then become the series expert on Sky's *Killing Mum and Dad* documentaries and there had been a number of other TV appearances since then.

But these were brief commentaries; I was a forensic psychologist, not a celebrity. And I certainly didn't have a social media presence apart from my own very private account on Facebook. I still thought that trolls were the hairy things that lived under bridges in fairy tales. Work had always flowed in via word of mouth, so I didn't need to promote myself with a website. And if I did, I had always thought that I would be the one to decide on its content.

I wrote back immediately, politely thanking him for his wholly unsolicited offering. I even said I was flattered – I wasn't remotely, I was creeped out, but such was my female programming to placate and be well-mannered that I said it all the same. I made it clear I was extremely uncomfortable with anybody creating a website for me but that as a gesture of goodwill I would reimburse him for the domain names, which a little bit of research revealed would have cost him around £20.

His reply pinged back almost immediately, his tone now flipped from vaguely polite to something altogether more terse and sinister:

'I could continue to run it as a fan or tribute site but I'm not sure that I want to be psychoanalysed. I don't see anything illegal in carrying on but in order to save any embarrassment or legal proceedings etc, I will sell the domain name to you for £3000.'

Clearly, I wasn't going to be buying anything from this pushy salesman. I reiterated my request that he remove the website, decided not to engage any further and left it at that. But the following week when I looked online to see if it had been taken down, I instead saw a site that was very much still standing and read the hateful words that I was now staring at in disbelief.

Online abuse is now a depressingly everyday part of life for women, especially those in the public eye. A 2017 study by Amnesty International clarified what any woman with a Twitter handle already knows. Online abuse of women is widespread, with one in five women suffering some kind of harassment, much of it sexually or physically threatening. The 'online' bit is something of a red herring, because the effects of the abuse are experienced offline, with over half of those surveyed reporting increased anxiety, panic attacks and stress as a result of the 'virtual' abuse, as well as other psychological consequences like loss of self-esteem and a sense of powerlessness. Amnesty's 'troll patrol' counted over a million abusive tweets alone sent to the women in the study over the course of 2017 — that's one every 30 seconds. The outlook gets even worse if you are a black or ethnic minority woman, and/or LGBTQ.

This was still the comparatively early days of the internet and there wasn't the same awareness around the perils of simply being a woman online. The idea that someone you'd never seen or met before could intimidate you from the anonymous comfort of their living room hadn't yet been declared an occupational hazard of being female. I watched with a strange vibration inside my chest as each day new 'content' went up on his site.

There were sexually graphic comments that made specific references to my clothing, especially a pair of jeans I wore when off-duty. I didn't take his sartorial critique too much to heart, but it did occur to me that I never wore jeans on TV and I'm usually filmed from the waist up – a talking head, not a talking bottom (although some may beg to differ). He must have seen me wearing them in real life. I was being stalked.

Lawmakers are usually more than a few steps behind trends in crime. Upskirting – the act of secretly filming or taking a photo under a woman's clothes – became illegal in England and Wales in 2019, but only after an 18-month campaign by Gina Martin, who was photographed unawares at a music festival. Back in 2011, the Protection from Harassment Act was in place, but it didn't specifically name or define stalking as a criminal offence. The government didn't introduce the crimes of stalking and stalking involving a fear of violence until November 2012. This followed research that found that one in five women and one in ten men will experience stalking in their adult life and a parliamentary inquiry making clear that the law was inadequate, the training of professionals piecemeal and victims' advocacy non-existent. The factor that differentiates stalking from harassment is the persistent, determined and altogether obsessive nature of the unwanted attention, something the existing laws didn't address.

Friends and relatives of targets can also often find themselves drawn into a stalker's preoccupation. While I was tackling this strange website, my sister, who was on Twitter long before me, received some tweets from an anonymous account. One said: 'Your sister is a vile disgusting bitch.' Another declared: 'Your sister is pathetic. No wonder she is divorced. Who would date a shrink like that? Hideous.'

I've never been married, but I was briefly engaged, in 2009, to a criminal law barrister who kept his wig in a Batman lunchbox. We'd given the appropriate notice at the register office near my home, but rather than live unhappily ever after we cancelled the wedding and went our separate ways. Information about my non-starter nuptials could only have been gleaned by searching public records; this person had discovered that I was not married now, but failed to join the dots correctly and assumed that I must be divorced. He knew I was single and probably that, apart from my cat Bijou, I was living alone.

He later went on to write outrageous and false allegations about my work online. He said that I was not a bona fide forensic psychologist, and went as far as calling me a criminal. I later discovered this was because he'd found evidence of a £100 fine I'd paid for filing my tax return late – I was hardly in line for an Interpol red notice. Had he gone through my bins (and that is not beyond the realms of possibility) he might have also discovered that I am not as fastidious with my recycling as I should be. That is how despicable I really am.

He frequently urged his readers to 'stay tuned' and promised to reveal the truth about the real me in his forthcoming biography of my life: 'The Devil You Don't Know'.

These rambling slurs on my name were far more galling for me than any of the comments about the shape of my body. To have my hard-won professionalism and integrity called into question by someone I'd never met felt like a sort of virtual poison. Even worse, I realized that if a site visitor contacted 'me' via this website they received a reply saying 'Thank you for contacting Kerry Daynes'. It was not inconceivable then that potential clients, solicitors, police officers, TV producers, even judges – anyone – could have emailed who they believed was 'me' via this site and I would not have known anything about it. Not only was I being stalked, but my career was now also under siege.

Clearly, and for reasons best known to him, this man was incredibly angry with me. Ostensibly, it was because I rejected his website proposal, but if it was a simple matter of business the slew of vicious and defamatory remarks would have served little purpose. And without a purpose, this behaviour could only exist to serve a much broader fury.

It's hard to capture how deeply unsettling it feels to realize that you have somehow awoken a random person's rage. Reading that kind of spite feels every bit as shocking as if it was said to your face, leaves you as winded as you would be by a physical blow.

Not knowing who this person was meant that anyone and everyone could potentially be him – the person walking behind me in the street or standing in the queue at the Post Office. I started to feel on edge when I went out, but equally didn't feel safe behind my own front door either, because he had explicitly mentioned on the website that he knew my address, commenting 'it isn't a difficult thing to get hold of'.

I had already tried calling the police.

They traced him through the details he had used to pay for the site registration and went to see him at his home, which it turned out was uncomfortably close to mine. But I didn't know they'd been to see him until I read about it on his website.

BREAKING NEWS – the police call at my home address.

…Talk about harassment from a female! They came around at Ms Daynes behest.

As it happened they only sent one officer so they obviously don't think I am high-risk…He asked if I was stalking Ms Daynes and I laughed out loud and said 'absolutely not…has she suggested I have?'

He asked if I would discontinue my websites and I said absolutely not. I welcome litigation by Ms Daynes. I told the officer Ms Daynes should be charged with wasting police time and she thinks all police are psychopaths…I assured him that Ms Daynes has nothing to fear from me of a criminal nature. He said 'you are absolutely right, the whole case is a civil matter.'

My stalker had given me a full report of his meeting with the police – rather than, as you would expect, the police themselves.

When I contacted the police they confirmed that, as far as they were concerned, no offence had been committed. It was, as he had said, a civil matter. It struck me then, as it does now, that the phrase 'a civil matter' is the stalking victim's equivalent of 'just a domestic' to a battered spouse.

I pointed to the fact that he clearly knew what clothes I had been wearing, had searched for my address online, and that he knew I was single and lived alone. He was making me feel threatened. But it was my job to provide evidence of this, they explained. Could I provide a log of his behaviour, even better could I get photographs of him watching me? It seemed like I had to turn stalker myself to catch my stalker. Except I had never seen him and had no idea what he looked like. How was I going to take photographs of him?

I felt incredibly let down by the police response – with inadequate laws and legislation to guide them, they had failed to see the bigger picture.

It was a horrible position to be in – and my insight as a forensic psychologist was proving more of a hindrance than a help. Stalking has been nicknamed 'assault in slow motion' because the drip-drip of stalking behaviours tends to escalate over time if left unchecked, and too frequently culminates in violence. I was only too aware that a high proportion of murders of women (94 per cent according to research conducted since then by the University of Gloucestershire) are preceded by stalking (surveillance activity, including covert watching, was recorded 63 per cent of the time by the same study). In short, not all stalkers are killers, but most killers of women start out as stalkers.

But I also knew that the risk is highest where a prior intimate relationship has existed between the stalker and the victim. And – even taking into account his fevered imagination – that clearly did not apply here. I tried to reassure myself with the rational, factual evidence that it was highly unlikely that a physical attack would happen to me. I knew that stalking by a stranger was likely to escalate into violence in roughly one in ten cases, rather than the 50 per cent of cases involving former partners. And I was a professional who had made a career out of working with, and keeping my cool around, high-risk men, after all.

And yet I also worked precisely where the unlikely existed. And I knew how unexpectedly and irreversibly things could escalate.

This was something my anxiety liked to remind me of at three in the morning, when it shook me awake and whispered to me: Are you safe? Are you *sure* you are safe? Are you *sure* you are sure? And then, the smallest and yet most fear-provoking question we ever ask ourselves: What if?

My mind returned more than once to a patient I had treated many years before, a young man who was plagued by a delusional belief that Chinese Triad members were trying to kill him. We spent a series of lengthy sessions testing the reality of his beliefs, reflecting sensibly on how the likelihood of him being killed by the gang was very low. I heard just a few weeks after his discharge from hospital that he had been shot dead by drug dealers in Manchester who, unbeknown to me, he owed money to. I was reminded of what

Joseph Heller wrote in *Catch 22*: 'Just because you're paranoid doesn't mean they aren't after you'.

I set about making my home a fortress, and upped the security with a new alarm system and extra locks. I even moved out for a while and went to stay with a friend, only moving back home when I got myself a giant dog – much to my cat's disgust, he had been king of the garden for 11 years by then. Humphrey joined Fozzchops a few months later. I'm not sure what my lionesque chow-chows would have done in the event of an intruder, but the size of them and their unrelenting loyalty were, and still are, a reassuring presence.

This was undoubtedly an unwelcome blurring of the line between work and home life that I had tried so assiduously to maintain over the years. And as used as I was to quashing my own gut reactions – pushing the eyeball to one side – it's fair to say that, for the first time in a long time, I was truly scared. Scared of a man. Scared of a man who I had never met and had never been involved with, physically or emotionally.

*

This all happened just a few weeks before I first met Liam, a man with a history of degrading attacks on women. So a sense of my gender being the touch paper for a dose of misogynist vitriol was at the front of my mind during the weeks I spent with him.

The first time Liam went to prison he was just 18

years old. His girlfriend, who was 17 and petite, with long blonde hair, had laughed at him for being clumsy during foreplay; the pair were at her parents' house messing about on the sofa. So he punched her in the face, stripped her naked, tied her arms to a dining chair and beat her repeatedly across her body with the buckle end of his belt. He left her there in the middle of the room, in a state of shock, attaching her legs to the chair before he left so that her genitals were on display to whoever came home and found her.

After his release for that attack he spent three blemish-free years on the outside but was arrested again, this time after assaulting another slightly built, blonde teenage girl. He had followed her home from the pub she worked at as a glass collector, a route which took in a shortcut across a disused children's play area in the middle of a residential estate. He came up behind her and 'blitz' attacked her: punched her in the back of the head, kicked her feet out from under her so she fell down to the ground and stamped on her. He knelt next to her and masturbated over her, while she was semi-conscious, before running off.

Unfortunately for him she had been more conscious than he realized and she was able to identify him as a recent regular of the pub. In fact she had noticed him a couple of times while she had been out shopping, but thought nothing of it. When he was arrested, police found detailed notes about her shift patterns, the clothes she wore plus the movements of two other girls – the same age, the same small frame and fair colouring – along with pictures he'd drawn of girls, bound and naked, being kicked or punched. They were cartoon images, quite accomplished, enlarged heads with distressed faces and droplets of sweat spraying outwards from them. Laced-up boots and disembodied fists coming down on them. Liam's criminal behaviour was an ugly caricature in every sense. It is not that often that a case file includes a fully illustrated guide to the fantasy life and offence rehearsals of a predatory stalker.

The Stalking Risk Profile, developed over the course of 20 years by leading psychologists and psychiatrists in the field, assigns stalking offenders to five different motivational types. Liam's behaviour was definitely true to type for the rarest of the bunch: a predatory stalker. These are men who follow and collect information about their victim, typically a female and a stranger to them, as an elaborate precursor to a violent or sexual assault. For this stalker type, the sense of excitement and anticipation that comes from covertly watching an unsuspecting victim is as gratifying as the ultimate attack.

Far more typical than predatory or other types is the rejected stalker, someone who is either attempting to reconcile with a former intimate partner, or seeking revenge for the rejection they have suffered when the relationship ended or they were rebuffed. Other types include the incompetent suitor who targets strangers or acquaintances, and is driven by a combination of lust and loneliness, going entirely the wrong way about trying to lure their victim into a brief encounter such as a date or a short-term sexual liaison. The intimacy-seeking stalker is fuelled by delusional beliefs that they are already in an intense relationship with the victim. And the resentful stalker blazes with the conviction that they have been mistreated or humiliated by their target, and wants to settle the score. While useful as guideline indicators of behaviour, what drives a stalker's behaviour is often complex and shifting. He or she won't necessarily behave within the strict confines of one 'type' forever.

*

I was set to meet Liam at what is known as a forensic step-down service. 'Step-down service' sounds like a support group for someone who has recently retired from an illustrious career as the head of a major business empire, but in fact it's a place for former offenders who need extra help, or who need overseeing, in the transition from prison or (more often) secure hospital back into the real world. It's a halfway house, usually for those who might need more support than others, people with multiple or complex problems or drug dependencies, or those considered to have a high risk of reoffending.

I have always thought that anyone transferring out of

a prison into a step-down project is incredibly fortunate – although they may not necessarily always agree. Moving in is very different to finding yourself blinking in the daylight on the outside of the prison gates, all your worldly goods in hand and nowhere to go next. It is a supportive and effective environment – projects often have their roots in the church, with high ideals and an emphasis on making a valuable contribution to society. There is guidance with education and employment, often access to therapy and counselling, and a general steer in readjusting to the real world. But there are also restrictions, which might include a locked room at night, curfews and other strict parameters which the step-down resident needs to observe.

Ex-offenders who live in step-down services are more often than not managed by a MAPPA (multi-agency public protection arrangement) team. This involves input from the police, the probation services and the managers of the step-down project, who continually assess the risk a person might pose and do their best to keep everyone safe by adjusting the level of monitoring and restrictions placed on them accordingly. It isn't easy to be a member of the MAPPA – as a group you can only manage the likelihood of someone committing a crime through the limited powers of each agency, and decision making is often fraught with conflict and dilemmas.

Liam was referred to me after he had asked for some

of his restrictions to be lifted. He'd been living at the project for the last seven months without contention and had been peacefully and successfully sharing an annexe – a purpose-built extension at the back of a big Edwardian house – with five other men.

All the standard, detailed risk assessments had been completed by his MAPPA team, but before they handed him more freedom they felt that one last assessment was outstanding. The Psychopathy Checklist, also known as the PCL-R, or as Jon Ronson described it in his bestselling book, 'The Psychopath Test'. Ronson's paraphrasing title is a misnomer though, because strictly speaking the PCL-R isn't really a test at all.

It's a personality profiling process, developed in 1991 by Canadian researcher Dr Robert Hare. It identifies the extent to which a person demonstrates the 20 qualities of a psychopath and provides a sliding scale of psychopathy that all but the most virtuous of us are likely to fall on somewhere. Based on extensive interviewing and tooth-combing of file information, the person conducting the assessment – who must be a specially trained and qualified psychologist – scores each characteristic between zero and two, depending on whether it is present, partially present or absent. The maximum score possible therefore is 40, although to score 30 or more is to earn the dubious label of psychopath, and probably find you are never invited to dinner among polite society again.

The PCL-R groups the defining characteristics of a psychopath under two broad themes: personality traits and lifestyle factors. The former includes grandiosity, manipulativeness, indications of recklessness and a lack of concern for others. Traits which are undeniably unpleasant but shared by all manner of people, particularly those who actively seek out and thrive in the public gaze, such as celebrities, politicians and, according to one 2016 study, one-fifth of all corporate executives. Hare famously said that if he couldn't have studied psychopaths in prison settings, he would have studied stockbrokers or telemarketers instead. The lifestyle characteristics of the PCL-R address a person's track record for non-conformity, their propensity for breaking rules, commitments and the occasional heart. Points are scored for criminal behaviours including juvenile delinquency, engaging in a variety of different offence types and a history of breaking legal conditions or parole.

Although considered a gold standard assessment in forensic psychology, the PCL-R is also the subject of much debate. The problem is that what was conceived by Hare as a measure of personality and nothing more, has been repurposed, packaged up and commercialized to the extent that it is now widely used as an all-too-conclusive violence risk-assessment tool, meaning its results can have profound and long-lasting impacts on those who are expected to take it. In fact, it is only the few specific items on the PCL-R that measure a person's past criminal record that predict future offending and are therefore relevant to risk assessment. Opponents argue that the PCL-R is by no means an exhaustive examination of an individual, and that the concept of 'psychopathy' within this context is too simplistically circular: someone has done bad things and so that qualifies them as a psychopath, and if they're a psychopath ergo they'll do bad things.

Put simply it can sometimes seem like the tail wagging the dog, and me being asked to carry out that particular investigation at the step-down project was a case in point. I didn't feel it was going to add very much by way of assessing Liam's risk, given that he had already undergone a number of other risk assessments. In terms of his criminal behaviours, it would only tell us what we already knew about Liam's past. Also, taking into account that he had spent large chunks of his adult life so far in prison, he simply hadn't had the opportunities to amass the kind of curriculum vitae that's needed for a high score on the PCL-R.

But I had been asked to do it and the rationale of the PCL-R was not up for discussion at the time. Like so much forensic psychology, completing this job was about due process and ticking boxes – getting on with doing, not thinking. But I knew that Liam's MAPPA team were being thorough and I am all for being thorough, so I went along to meet him.

*

The step-down project was in a converted house and there were no meeting rooms or private spaces, so I waited for Liam in the communal kitchen. It was like any regular domestic kitchen except perhaps unusually clean, and peppered with giveaways like the notes above the plug sockets saying 'Do Not Unplug', the fire blankets on the wall and the rota for kitchen cleaning duties on the back of the door. Blue fitted cupboards clad the walls, punctuated by a large window overlooking the garden that was plotted out allotment-style – a scheme to keep residents busy.

I was looking out over the garden when Liam walked in, and when I turned around to greet him I noticed him obviously look me up-and-down, taking in my figure before he got to my face. This is something that most women experience at some point, but despite it being familiar I still take notice when it happens, not only for the cheek of it, but for the deeper, more telling indication that, for the man in question, clocking-up a woman's vital statistics is the priority in this situation.

He didn't smile at me and only just managed to shake my hand rather limply before he pulled his chair out and sat down, elbows on the table and fingers clasped together in front of his face. He was uncomfortable and irritated.

But I could understand that – who greets the news that they are doing a 'psychopath test' with good humour?

Having done the introductions I conducted my own, less transparent, brief physical assessment of him – a man now in his late 30s, medium height and build, wearing jeans and a plain black sweatshirt. He was unremarkable in almost every way, his hair shaved short at the back and sides, a slackness in his shoulders and the pallor of someone who doesn't get out much.

I explained the PCL-R, reassured him that it is a widely used forensic assessment, and asked him if he had any questions. He said he just wanted to get on with it. And added that it was about time it was done, because he wanted his restrictions lifted. For a moment I felt like a travel agent dealing with an unhappy holidaymaker who was complaining because his room didn't have a view. His sense of entitlement seemed bold, and out of context here.

But he was right, his restrictions were tight. His room was locked and alarmed at night and he wasn't able to leave the house without consent from the manager. If he did go out he was required to stick to his work placements and probation appointments, and to central, densely populated areas of the town centre. He also had to produce evidence of where he had been in the form of receipts and bus tickets. This is by no means solid proof of someone's movements, but is part of a mutual trust-building ethos which the step-down resident should ideally be keen to comply with.

We began the process. The PCL–R interview schedule isn't something that can be quickly filled out on an A4 clipboard. It's a lengthy and protracted process, a green paper booklet with pages of prompts and probes designed to gather information about everything from family background and intimate relationships to financial matters and criminal activities. It can take a number of hours to get through, and is best done over a period of days. The nature of the conversations you have, and all the additional information you gather along the way, mean it's a deeply involved and intense experience for both the interviewee and the person asking the questions. I knew I'd be visiting Liam there over a number of weeks.

Liam settled into the interviews quite quickly but his answers were on the brief side. I felt he was giving me as much information as I probed for and nothing more. The idea is to make the conversation feel as natural and unforced as possible, but I was struggling to gain any sort of rapport. He didn't want to work with me and looked at me throughout in a way that said, Come on then woman, get on with it. He was scoring a big fat zero on item one of the checklist: superficial charm.

(Superficial charm is one of the 20 characteristics of the PCL–R, but that doesn't mean that an individual with an overall high score will automatically get points here. I have found that the further north of the country I go the less likely a client is to score highly on this. In fact, my favourite research study of all time investigated why Scottish criminals scored less on the PCL–R than their American counterparts. Investigators found it was because they lack the Americans' glib, charming manners! American psychopaths tell you to 'Have a nice day', Scottish ones, not so much.)

With no designated meeting rooms in the house it was a case of pitching our tent where we could, so we mostly sat in the communal lounge area on the shabby chenille sofas, a fish tank full of multicoloured guppies gulping away behind Liam as I talked to him over the coffee table, which was sticky with the overspill of a hundred mugs of sweet tea. It felt like a two-star guesthouse – something that might come up on one of those reality TV shows about shoddy hospitality. We didn't get any peace, either. The radio was on and other residents would come and go, switch on the TV, feed the fish, ask if we had any cigarettes.

I wasn't jumping to any conclusions but I felt fairly certain his score wasn't going to indicate an unusually high psychopathy level. I would need to make my final calculations, but experience told me that his final score was going to be in the region of 15–18 out of a possible 40. Your average score for a prison inmate is between 19 and 22; your typical man or woman in the street, unless they are Mary Poppins, tends to score between 3 and 6 (my own score, if I am brutal with myself, is 4).

After our penultimate session I thought I'd take a second look through Liam's file documentation. That's when I remembered the collection of receipts and travel tickets and asked to see them. They might tell me more about this brusque man and what he did in his free time and, as I said, I'm all for being thorough. What I saw made the hairs on the back of my neck start to prickle.

The seemingly innocuous paperwork of someone's daily life has much to tell, particularly when it is presented and filed in chronological order. Patterns emerge and personal preferences quickly become clear. There was a thick bundle of receipts, held together with a yellow elastic band and I began to thumb through them, like the pages of a flicker book, the picture emerging unexpectedly. We knew Liam went into town most days and that he was expected to stay in the busy part of the shopping centre. His receipts showed that he bought bread for the project on Wednesdays, he bought a monthly angling magazine and often bought mints at the same stationers, before heading straight to the same Costa Coffee, a busy cafe with the kind of two-person counter service where one person stays on the till and the other makes the coffees and serves them further down the counter. Liam's receipts showed that over time – a period of a few months – he had begun to visit the Costa exclusively on the same days – always Thursday and Friday afternoons and any time on Saturday. Sometimes he went in there as many as three or four times on the same day. He always had the same drink – a cappuccino – and I noticed from the name on the receipt that it was almost always the same person who served him: Esther.

I didn't say anything to Liam about it when I saw him and we worked through what were the final sections of the PCL-R interview quite quickly. Afterwards I used the staff computer to type up my notes, then had a look online to see where the coffee shop was, thinking that maybe I'd pop in there. The feeling that Liam's commitment to this branch of Costa might be driven by something more than an appreciation of their cappuccinos was weighing on my mind. While I was searching the shopping centre website, an advert for a well-known men's deodorant popped up in the sidebar, showing a woman bent seductively over an oven. The strap-line read 'Can she make you lose control?'

I looked at the time on the screen – it was lunchtime. I decided to take a stroll into town. This wasn't an especially extraordinary thing to do, I had to eat after all, but it also seemed like a good opportunity to walk in Liam's shoes for a moment.

*

On the short walk down the pedestrianized shopping street to Costa I passed a pretty blonde teenager. She was wearing headphones and was dressed in a school uniform that she had tried to make as non-school-uniform as possible. I remembered my own days as a self-conscious schoolgirl – far too keen to grow up – and I smiled at her as she walked past.

She didn't smile back. I got the kind of blank, mildly disdainful look you get from teenagers who are listening to music and have no interest in you, which was healthy as far as I was concerned. But it got me thinking about how a look like that would be interpreted by Liam and, yes, by my own stalker. What would they feel or see in that brief exchange? Would that smile rebuffed, that slightest of rejections, inflame their anger?

How dangerous people are at any given time in their lives depends on a wide range of elements, not least the situation in which they find themselves. If Liam felt the girl slighted him I knew it would have stoked his loathing, because in this scenario she was in the unfortunate position of being both coveted and loathed. He wanted to be desired and felt entitled to be obeyed, but if he felt rejection and perhaps ridicule his veins would begin to course with resentment: She thinks she is better than me.

I wondered if his mind would have taken him back momentarily to previous attacks and he would have reimagined the pain he had seen and savoured – his victims' bodies powerless, their faces terrified and humiliated. He had wanted them to feel his power, his anger, and to pay. I recalled how, in the PCL-R interview, I had asked him about how he felt in the moment he had attacked his girlfriend. He didn't know what he was thinking, he said, only rage and the need to stop her from laughing at him, looking down at him, insulting him. That had sent him 'berserk'. But he felt calmer afterwards, he said. The payback had been satisfying.

In a situation like this, a crowded high street in the middle of the day, that kind of rage wouldn't be able to reach such a climax without attracting attention; there were no isolated spots, his options were limited. But it would still bubble away, under the surface.

I opened the door to the cafe, the warm air and smell of coffee and Danish pastries wafting over me. I picked up a sandwich from the fridge and a bottle of water and joined the small queue to pay. The girl at the counter asked if I wanted anything else but I was too busy looking at her name badge to hear her the first time: it was Esther, a short girl with fair hair in a ponytail, she looked about 17.

*

The next week I was at the step-down again to brief Sheila the project manager and Liam on the results of his PCL-R assessment. As predicted, he had a fairly average score, there was nothing screaming psychopath. It didn't warrant balloons and a congratulations card, but it was at least something mildly positive to start with – no psychopath sticker today!

But the tone quickly darkened when I said I had, however, found something that gave me cause for concern and was relevant to the likelihood of his reoffending. I laid out the bundle of receipts from his trips to the coffee shop on the table between us – well over 100 of them – and said, treading the line somewhere between non-accusatory and firm: 'I've noticed that you visit this cafe when a particular girl is on shift. I would really like to get your take on this, Liam.'

Instantly, his eyebrows came together like a pair of curtains and his mouth fell into a flat, hard line. Then he pointed at me and spat: 'You fucking bitch.'

Sheila and I glanced briefly at each other and then back to Liam. We didn't say anything.

'Jesus Christ. Since when has buying a coffee been a fucking crime? You're fucking warped.'

Then, more to himself than me: 'Fucking bitches.'

I lowered my voice slightly. 'It's not a crime to buy coffee, Liam, but I wouldn't be doing my job properly if I didn't ask about this. I am concerned for the safety of this woman and I want to help you too. I think it would be helpful to talk about it so that we can understand what is going on for you. What do you think?'

Liam stood up and swept his hand across the table, sending the pile of receipts – now back in their elastic band – flying. Instinctively I put my hand out and somehow managed to catch them. He leant down on both arms and his eyes tightened into a glare. 'I think you are an interfering old whore,' he said. His lip curled into a contemptuous snarl. 'I wouldn't even touch you.' He kicked the leg of the table, and stormed out of the room.

There was silence as we held our breath for a couple of beats, then Sheila and I looked at each other. 'Right then,' I said. 'That went well.'

She nodded her head towards the papers in my left hand. 'Good save.'

I heard from her later that his MAPPA team, upon reading my report and recommendations, had decided that Liam's restrictions were not going to be lifted any time soon.

*

LITIGATION BECKONS:

I will publish all correspondence from Ms Daynes' solicitors…unfortunately for Ms Daynes this will only further damage her reputation.

I am prepared to make an offer to Ms Daynes to settle out of court. In view of time and effort, personal grievance and damage to my own reputation I will accept £5000 from her in full and final settlement. In satisfaction of this I will remove the website.

A couple of months after working with Liam I found myself at the Manchester Civil Justice Centre, a modern, light-filled court which seemed to add to the strangeness of the day. I was more at home with the Victorian Gothic style of the Crown Court down the road, where the wood panelling and ornate carvings seemed to lend a seriousness to the proceedings that I missed here in this airy, wide-open space.

I sat, flanked by my legal team, and saw for the first time the man behind the website. It had dawned on me as he walked into the court that this was the same innocuous-looking person who had, just a few minutes ago, been sitting a few feet away from me in the cafe downstairs. I didn't give him the satisfaction of a single moment of eye contact – I knew he would already be luxuriating in this grand day out with me. As he took his seat in front of me I noticed a thread had come loose on the seam on the back of his light blue suit.

We had pursued him for defamation and libel, to get his website taken down. There was also a very real possibility that clients could mistakenly send sensitive and potentially explosive material to him and I had a duty of care to them not to let that happen. I really had been given no other option than to take it to court, thus making it a 'civil matter'.

He was ordered to convert his website to a blank white screen and destroy any and all material relating to me. Then came the question of my legal bill. Civil proceedings don't come cheap, meaning that protecting yourself from a stalker's barrage by this route isn't something everyone can afford.

The judge asked him to stand up: 'Do you have £60,000 to pay Miss Daynes' costs?'

He started to become flustered and said, 'Well I wouldn't relish it,' alluding to what was clearly wishful thinking that he had it but just didn't fancy parting with it.

However, I knew then that I would not be pursuing him for the recovery of my costs. He was representing himself and had incurred no fees other than the cost of his own time. He'd also been keen to try to charge me for his websites throughout this whole episode. It didn't seem like he had any money. You can't get blood out of a stone. And truth be told, I didn't have any inclination to go after this presumably already deeply unhappy man. Doing so would only maintain a perverse sort of connection to him.

The judge continued: 'Do you understand that Miss Daynes does not want any form of business relationship with you? She does not want any other form of relationship with you. Do you understand that she has not made any form of voluntary contact with you?'

And that is when he said: 'It doesn't matter because I'm finished with her now, I'm done with her. She upset me.' As if we'd had a promising romance which had suddenly turned sour.

I exchanged glances with the legal assistant on my left. My solicitor, sitting on my right, picked up his blue biro and discreetly opened his ring binder. He scribbled something, then positioned the folder in a way that I could read it, before closing it again.

He had written the word: 'NUTTER'.

I smiled weakly and then fixed my gaze again on the errant thread on the back of my adversary's jacket. He wasn't a 'nutter' (whatever that meant) any more than Liam was a 'psychopath'. In my mind's eye, I crossed out the word on the paper and then replaced it, in large, red imaginary letters, with the word 'misogynist'.

Misogyny – an ingrained prejudice against and contempt for women and girls – is one of the few human conditions that hasn't yet been declared a mental illness. Probably because, if it were, it would be a pandemic. In the courtroom that day it seemed clear to me that here was just another of misogyny's foot soldiers: a man who resented a woman's rejection so much that he wanted to punish her for it.

I walked out of court that day a lot poorer, but feeling relief that I had at least tackled a problem head-on. It was over. I went home, switched the alarm off as I opened the door, closed my curtains and went to lie down on my sofa. The strain of the day had triggered a Ménière's attack and I knew it would be ferocious. The room began to turn. But as I lay there with Fozzchops snoring loudly at my feet, I reassured myself that at least one situation was no longer spinning out of control.

Or so I thought. I couldn't have imagined then that I would still be dealing with it six years later. In this job you have to get used to unfinished stories.

CHAPTER 9
THE CASE OF THE MISSING FINGER

If I can't stay where I am, and I can't,
then I will put all that I can into the going.
Jeanette Winterson, *Why Be Happy When You Could*
Be Normal?

By May 2013 austerity had well and truly hit. Cost-cutting measures, administered in the wake of the 2008 global financial crisis, were applied to public sector services with the sting of military-issue iodine.

The Ministry of Justice was seeing its overall budget shrink by 40 per cent – among the deepest cuts to any government department. A huge slash in spending on Legal Aid meant my work as an expert witness in the courts had almost disappeared (it seems experts are non-essential when money is tight. Although given the increasing number of people appearing in criminal and family courts without even legal advice or representation, the demise of psychologists sounds trifling). Contracts that I had with charities, social care organizations and local authorities had all been cut or put out to tender and won by cheaper providers – volunteer counsellors, trainees or, even worse, life coaches. I was being asked to train fewer police officers, being consulted less frequently on interrogations and investigations. I had always told my clients that crime doesn't pay and it was proving true for me now – requests for my services were very much down.

Except in one area. Due in part to Operation Yewtree, the investigation into child abuse committed by former TV personality Jimmy Savile among others, there had been a wave of public awareness of and confidence in reporting child abuse offences. The number of arrests and subsequent prosecutions wasn't rising anywhere near as fast as the disclosure rate. But, that said, in my practice demand for pre-sentence reports about sex offenders who had committed internet-based crimes against children were unremitting. Referrals came in weekly from solicitors whose clients were men who'd been found downloading child abuse imagery online (there is and never has been any such thing as 'child pornography' – just child abuse and pictures, videos and even, as I was learning, livestreaming of it). A proportion of these included those who had incited children to engage in sexual conversations or activity via chatrooms and webcams, or had attempted to meet up with them. They were mostly older men, but sometimes also younger, in their late teens and early 20s, boys who had learned the art of 'grooming' (the process by which an abuser manipulates a victim and overcomes any likely resistance by them over time) via their own experience of having been exploited online as children. Young or old, there was rarely anything outwardly unusual about any of them, they held down jobs, were in relationships and had little history of rule-breaking.

Their files usually included a case summary giving three or four sample descriptions of the material that had been retrieved from their mobile phones and computers. Every image is assessed and categorized according to the severity of the abuse involved, the spectrum running from children photographed in sexualized poses through to footage of the most extreme and brutal acts.

In 2013 a five-point grading scale was in use (known as the SAP scale; it has since been replaced by a simpler three-tier system introduced by the Sentencing Council). I always felt for the specialist officer whose job it had been to view the image, assign it to a category, catalogue it and type up the summary, the language always so remote and formal, yet unable to disguise the horror of what it detailed. I found having to read them every day hard enough to cope with. It wasn't only the graphic accounts of what these adults had done to children that I was finding hard to process, but the sheer number of abusive images in circulation. That, and the one detail that the summary description never tells you: whether the child had been identified and was safe now, or still out there somewhere being subject to more of the same.

The National Crime Agency estimates there are up to 80,000 people in the UK who 'present some kind of sexual threat' to children online. Increasingly, it felt to me as though all of them were on my caseload (the only more disturbing thought being that they weren't on anybody's caseload). The varied and unpredictable nature of my work and clients had always been one of the things I loved most about forensic psychology. I didn't want to strike a whole tranche of offenders from my list, but at the same time my head was brimming with unwanted, half-imagined images and I was beginning to feel quite strongly that I hadn't signed up for this.

It was around this time that I was asked by BBC Wales to contribute to a Welsh-language documentary. I had deliberately stayed out of the public eye since being stalked – keeping a low profile felt the safest thing to do – and had turned down a number of documentaries. The stalker appeared to be a sleeping dog and I was happy to let him lie. But on this occasion I took a punt on the fact that he probably wasn't that fluent in Welsh so wouldn't be watching, and said yes.

They wanted me to contribute to a film covering the trial of Mark Bridger. Wales had been in mourning since the previous autumn, when five-year-old April Jones, who had cerebral palsy, was abducted and murdered by Bridger. Her disappearance while out playing sparked the biggest missing person search in UK police history. Not only did Bridger kill her, he disposed of her body in such a way that she has never been found. He incinerated parts of her body in the wood burner at his home, but forensic teams found tiny particles of skull in the fireplace and bloodstains matching April's DNA. It is believed that he scattered other parts of her in the countryside and possibly in the fast-running river near his cottage in Ceinws. April's parents were only ever able to bury 17 fragments of their daughter's remains.

Bridger pleaded not guilty to the charge of murdering April, but accepted that he was 'probably responsible' for her death. The mystery of what had happened to this little girl, the lack of closure that the discovery of her body or a coherent explanation by Bridger might have given, contributed to a deluge of media interest in the case, and in the evidence that might emerge during his trial.

I had been asked to watch as Bridger gave his evidence and to provide some commentary to the filmmakers. I took my seat in the narrow press and public mezzanine of Mold Crown Court for a week, fully expecting to watch events play out with the same impartial interest I had always cultivated at work. But it was the first time I'd seen anything like this from that viewpoint: high up, in the same room and yet light years away from the people whose fate is being decided below. I wasn't an expert witness there to give my opinion and I wasn't the victim there to see justice served. I found that I could only watch and absorb as any other member of the public might, in turns appalled by the grotesque charade Bridger played out and humbled by the quiet dignity and strength of April's parents.

It was a few seconds of video that got me, the CCTV footage of her in the leisure centre on the day he took her, a happy, unusually small girl struggling to open a heavy door by herself. And there he was in court, a six-foot-two man, the snake tattoo on his forearm covered by a blue shirt. Later that day she would become fragments of bone in his fireplace. Watching that clip I felt an anger rise in me, and knew it wasn't going anywhere soon.

We heard how, in the days before he took April, Bridger had been searching the internet for images of Soham murder victims Holly Wells and Jessica Chapman, and the schoolgirl Caroline Dickinson who was raped and killed on a school trip to France in 1996. We were told about files on his computer containing obscene imagery of child abuse. Other searches on his computer included words like 'puberty' and 'naked young five year old'.

Bridger protested that he had been doing internet research to understand his own children's sexual development. He had saved indecent images of children 'to complain about them later', he insisted. He said he accidentally ran over April in his Land Rover and that he was unable to fully recall what had happened next because he was drunk and in a state of panic. But we then heard an eight-year-old witness testify that she had seen April climbing into his car. Forensic scientist Roderick Stewart told the jury that there was not a trace of physical evidence, either on Bridger's Land Rover or on April's bike, to back up his claim that there had been an accident.

It was obvious to everyone what he had been fantasizing about before he abducted April, there was really no question that he had killed her and that the crime was sexually motivated. It even emerged that he had tried and failed to get three other girls into his car that day. His lies were risible and calculated, and it seemed to me his cruelty in withholding from her parents the truth of what happened was impossible to forgive.

On 30 May, Bridger was found guilty of abduction, murder and perverting the course of justice. He was sentenced to life imprisonment with a whole-life tariff. It has long been my view that if you take a child's life then the only rightful place for you to end your life is a prison. But I'm not paid to make judgements of that kind. And until then I had always somehow managed to compartmentalize my personal feelings about someone's offending behaviour so that I was able to work with them objectively, considering the person as well as the offence. I'd met more than anybody's share of child killers in prisons, including Robert Black, who was responsible for the death of at least four girls (and who died in HMP Maghaberry in 2016). I'd also worked with several men in forensic step-down services who were moving on from jail terms for abducting or killing children. I would introduce myself and offer them my hand when I met them, just as I would with anyone else, and think only of the job in hand, not their hand in mine.

Apart from Ian Brady (you don't grow up in Manchester and later shake Ian Brady's hand without thinking of the harm that hand has caused), did I feel revulsion? Yes. But I also still managed to find a shred of compassion for Brady. What a wretched soul, I remember thinking to myself. But over those days as I listened to Mark Bridger repeatedly referring to the child he had killed as 'little April', I knew that I couldn't find the detachment I needed to feel neutral about him. I had never looked at somebody like I looked at Mark Bridger and felt so utterly repelled and disgusted.

During that week watching Bridger's testimony a colleague suggested I had 'post-traumatic stress disorder'. Perhaps I was suffering some kind of vicarious trauma that my standard supervision meetings with a fellow psychologist – all psychologists are required to take this time to offload and reflect on their work – weren't enough to help. I remember thinking that if PTSD meant 'permanently tired, sick and disgusted' then yes, I had a bout of that for sure. I had a caseload brimming with men who looked at images of children being abused and although they weren't all Mark Bridgers they were still part of it, buyers and traders in a thriving black market.

I gave my analysis of Bridger to the TV crew in the professional manner expected of me. I added how, for nearly 50 years now we've all been told about 'stranger danger', mainly thanks to a 1971 government campaign, which was precipitated by the Moors murders and other high-profile child abductions in the 1960s. It is an outdated concept. Defining 'abduction' and 'stranger' in the context of homicide is no longer so straightforward. We tend to think of children being lured or snatched off the street but some of the more recent cases have involved a degree of grooming online prior to contact and murder. Even Mark Bridger was not a total stranger to April as one of his own children went to the same school as her. But, I reminded myself sitting in court, the reality is that child abductions are rare, those ending in homicide exceptionally so. They are the cases that come into the media spotlight exactly because they are the worst-case scenario. Less than half of child abductions are the work of strangers – 42 per cent according to a report, based on police data collected in 2011/12, by the charity Action Against Abduction. The approximate annual figure for under-16s taken by strangers, according to the same report, is 50, with 15 of them being sexually assaulted. Not that the low numbers involved make it any less shocking or impactful. There is some small comfort in the fact that the research also found that three out of every four abduction attempts fail.

When I left Wales and got home I still felt so angry. It was a bile, virulent and nasty. The anger didn't subside, it bubbled up in quiet moments and, increasingly, in the early hours of the morning where I would find myself wide awake. I had spent too long looking into the abyss, the dark crevices of the mind where bad things dwell and fester, and now it was gazing back into me.

*

I carried a general grumpy malaise around for weeks after the Bridger trial, one that no amount of dog-walking, my preferred method of mindfulness meditation, could seem to alleviate. I knew my objectivity was under strain and for a forensic psychologist that's a big deal; a tightrope walker who has missed their step and may or may not take the next one. Although perhaps I wasn't yet ready to say it out loud, I was having doubts about my career and where it was going. Was I making any real difference? What did I want to do? Who did I want to be working with? I didn't have the answers but I did know that I was struggling with what I'd been left with.

I wasn't in a great mood that day at the hospital. It was a general hospital with male and female wards for acute psychiatry and the base for a raft of outpatient clinics, including complex care, psychiatry of substance misuse and learning disability. I'd been here more times than I could remember over the years, the disinfectant smell and the sounds of the place familiar and institutional.

I'd been here so many times, in fact, that I knew that the only half-decent thing to eat in the canteen was a jacket potato, so I headed straight there and picked up a tray, slamming it down a bit too hard on the runners around the front of the hot plates.

It wasn't quite lunchtime and the canteen was empty apart from me and an elderly man, still in his dressing gown and slippers, and his visitor. I slotted myself into the table furthest away from them, next to the window overlooking the car park. I just wanted to be alone with my subsidized potato and my existential crisis.

And then she sat down directly opposite me. Eating hadn't helped my mood at all and my immediate thought was simply: Oh. Get. *Lost.* There were rows of empty tables, each of them with an artificial gerbera flower in a pot and four perfectly good chairs, the moulded plastic ones with holes in that look like Connect 4 frames. She could have sat in any of them but had instead plonked herself in the one chair out of all the chairs that was closest to me. I looked away, trying to avoid eye contact.

She didn't get the hint at all and smiled and said, 'Hello.' She was in her 50s, her thin, light brown hair was short and her neck and shoulders were exposed by the summery dress she had on, the strapless kind with elasticated shirring around the top to keep it up. I noticed her bra strap was a grimy, indeterminate grey and digging into her flesh in a way that looked quite uncomfortable.

She grinned and said, 'Hello I'm Lucy,' and I just nodded my head, not wanting to give her the slightest hint that I might be willing to engage. The people over in the other corner got up and left and I was about to do the same. But she started talking to me.

I realized quite quickly that she might be learning-disabled and it made me stop for a second. I remembered what my mum had always said when I was young: if someone you don't know talks to you it might be the highlight of their day, the only conversation they may have.

She seemed harmless so I dug deep, took a big breath and made an effort to be kind. I arranged my face – another thing my mum still tells me to do – and stayed sitting there opposite her while she chatted away. She got up and came and sat directly next to me, and started to show me her jewellery. Her hands were stacked with heavy silver, the kind you get on the market with the incense and the dreamcatchers, rings all the way up her fingers, the skin underneath them green and a bit sweaty looking. That's when I noticed the finger. Her left-hand ring finger was shorter than the others – it was a stub, missing its top knuckle and the nail.

'What happened to your finger?' I asked. I'm no stranger to asking personal questions, something that was especially true at that particular time, when I was having to ask a lot of men about their masturbatory habits. But I felt unusually familiar myself that day; perhaps I had lost all sense of social convention because I was so burned out with it all. And she was so friendly.

'I cut it off,' she said.

The mental health worker in me automatically assumed it had been an act of self-harm and that some intolerable emotions must have overtaken her. 'What made you feel like doing that?' I asked.

Nothing really, she said, it was for her ex-boyfriend. He'd gone to prison and he had written to her saying that he wanted to be able to 'always keep a piece of her with him'. She had done as he suggested and cut her finger off for him so he could have it. He had been really romantic like that, she said.

That's when I remembered it – a disembodied finger that had been found while I was working as a locum at a prison, not long after I started out. Was this woman the owner of that withered digit from all those years ago?

It had been found by prison officers Wright and Aktar in a cell belonging to a prisoner named Fillingham. It was brown and all shrivelled, like something you find in the natural treats section of the pet shop. Although technically speaking it was a finger*tip*, the cut had been made just underneath the top knuckle, a three-centimetre stub from what looked like a ring or index finger. The nail was still there, still with the barest shimmer of pink polish on it. The colour reminded me of Avon's Iced Champink lipstick, a shade I wore as a teenager in the 80s, pearlized and a bit childish.

I'd been walking past Fillingham's cell that morning and glimpsed the pair of them hunched over the narrow desk, with the drawer open. A selection of items – socks, toothbrush, comb – were laid out on the grey wool blanket on the bed, in the kind of neat, systematic way I recognized as routine search procedure. Officers always work their way around clockwise from the cell door, checking over every piece of furniture and surface as they go. Fillingham would have been frisked and moved to another cell while they were doing the search.

Even in his 40s, Aktar could have passed for an adolescent, albeit one with some impressively dense dark facial hair. Wright was a broad slab of a bloke, younger than Aktar, only a few months out of training, and he was breathing heavily, looking quite nauseous. He was tugging on his tie and I wondered if he had forgotten that this part of his uniform is, for safety reasons, a clip-on.

I popped in to see what they were looking at so intently and then they showed me. I said: 'A finger?

Shit.' Not the most eloquent observation, but I hadn't come prepared for this development.

We all stood looking at the finger for a moment and then, for some reason, we all held out our hands and looked at our own fingers, like we were doing an audit.

The finger had fallen out of an apparently unopened packet of batteries, which on closer inspection had turned out to have been opened and resealed by someone keen to hide something. One of the batteries' innards had been taken out of its printed casing and the finger was hidden inside.

Fillingham possessed a full complement of fingers, so they knew it wasn't his, but he was notorious at the prison for being able to get hold of things. He was a kind of contraband corner shop. If you wanted some ink, Fillingham could knock you up a tattoo gun made from biro casings and radio batteries. Pornography, hooch (a prison homebrew made from fruit, sugar, bread and whatever else they can get their hands on) and even copies of the technical manuals used by prison psychologists. I'd heard that Fillingham offered coaching sessions to men who were due for parole board hearings. For a price, of course.

I'd heard he also had a particular fetish for collecting skin. He hoarded slivers of flesh from any inmate that was prepared to hand it over. He had all the prison self-harmers donating bits of themselves, and he was suspected of providing some of them with cutting tools.

Aktar sealed off the cell and I went to my meeting, carried on with my day. I heard that Fillingham denied all knowledge of it, invoking what I like to call the Shaggy Defence ('It wasn't me!'). As far as I knew, the finger had never been traced to an owner, in the prison or out, alive or dead. And now here was Lucy, sitting next to me in a corner of a hospital canteen.

'Oh, I understand,' I said, and she smiled, probably not accustomed to such casual acceptance of her explanation.

'How did you get it to him in prison?' I asked, saddened that she felt she needed to cut off a digit to prove her commitment to this man. A tragedy dressed up as romance.

She had wrapped it in clingfilm and put it in her knickers when she went to visit him, she said. Then when the guards were looking the other way she had passed it to him. She looked into the distance and raised her shoulders, wistful, as if she was remembering something beautiful.

How had she done it? Did she see a doctor to get it sewn up? Did no one think to ask where the missing piece had gone? I couldn't begin to ask her these questions because I didn't really want to know any more. The human mind likes to close a story; to mine, here was conclusion at last to the story that had started that day, 15 years earlier, in Fillingham's cell.

It was time for my meeting and I managed to extract myself from the corner she had me wedged in.

'My social worker says I'm vulnerable,' she said, almost as clarification, as I squeezed past her. And I felt that sadness again. Lucy had somehow come to believe she was at fault for being vulnerable. Why was the onus on her? She wasn't missing that finger because she was vulnerable, she had been coerced into chopping it off by someone who was willing to exploit her.

I told Lucy how much I had enjoyed meeting her – meaning every word – and told her to remember that there were plenty of men in the world but she'd only got nine and a half fingers, and she needed to look after them. She promised me she would.

As I put my tray on the stacker on the way out, old ham sandwiches and cold cups of tea spilling out of it, I felt I was also clearing away a different kind of mess. I knew I couldn't truly be certain that it was Lucy's finger in Fillingham's possession that day, but I was going to choose to believe it was, and that, in this resolution, a mystery had been solved. Not only the puzzling case of the finger, but the question of what I was going to do next.

It was time for me to take a break from frontline forensic psychology – from the sex offenders, and all the disillusionment I felt with the system I'd seen failing for so long. I would go to work in women's mainstream mental health services, where maybe I could help women like Lucy. The abyss I had been staring into was becoming a new horizon.

CHAPTER 10
SAFE AND SOUND

Denying emotion is not avoiding the high curbs, it's never taking your car out of the garage. It's safe in there, but you'll never go anywhere.
Brené Brown, *Rising Strong*

When she was eight years old, Maya had contracted scarlet fever. Although for most children the discomfort of such an illness – her throat ballooned and her body ached all over – would make for unpleasant memories, for Maya the experience of being sick was a revelation.

Confined to her bed, she had been cared for by her mother, who showed her a level of affection and attention that she'd never experienced before. Her dad had left her alone. More significant than this was the way she had been treated by the visiting doctor, a man she described as being 'like an angel'. She told me how he promised he would make her feel well again and had tucked her gently into bed. No one had ever done that before.

Her dad had been a gambler and a heavy drinker. If he wasn't home by 6pm in the evening everyone knew he'd gone to the pub and that they were in for a long night. Sometimes when he came home he would line the children up in a row – there were six of them, and he'd have to get the youngest out of bed – and hit each of them one by one, usually a punch in the stomach, so that the others could see what was coming to them next. He once punched Maya in the face so hard that it knocked her front teeth out. The scar was still visible on her adult face, a bright slash of fibrous tissue running from her nose to her lip.

Once, he poured a pot full of boiling rice over her mother's head when she wouldn't give him money. Another time, he had drowned the family cat's litter of new kittens in the bath, forcing Maya and her brothers and sisters to watch.

It was a reign of pure terror; callous violence administered by a man who took great pleasure in the theatre of his abuse. For most children a broken limb or even a fall from a bicycle is a big life event, something they remember all their lives because of just how much it hurt. Maya's father made sure his daughter spent large chunks of her childhood in fear and pain.

The moments she remembered feeling happy or secure were scant. The police were regular visitors to her home, she said, and she recalled the promises of an officer who had wrapped a blanket around her and reassured her that she would make things better, but had never come back. Another time, she and her siblings had moved out with their mother to a refuge and she made a friend there, Anne. She wished she had stayed in touch with Anne; she hadn't had such a friend since. But their father had found them, and life had very quickly furred over with its familiar sadness again.

*

It was my first job after my encounter with Lucy in the hospital canteen. I started to wind down and then closed my private practice. A few weeks later I started a new role as a consultant psychologist, within a private group of women's recovery hospitals. All of the facilities were small and homely, in discreet settings. This one, an old converted townhouse in a leafy residential street, innocuously located in a well-heeled North Manchester suburb, was a place where women who'd suffered major mental health episodes came to spend time and reacclimatize before making the transition back to their everyday lives. There were just six beds here and I had high hopes for what I was going to achieve in this kind of environment, it felt so welcoming and natural – a long way from the clinical interview rooms with fixed furniture and guards standing by that I knew from prisons, or the sterility of secure hospitals and wards. The doors of this hospital locked automatically behind you, but that was to keep the danger out, not the patients in.

So my heart sank when I discovered who the other fresh arrival to the hospital was. The nurse manager announced during morning handover that our new resident Maya was joining us with a diagnosis of 'erotomania' and a history of stalking. With my own experience of being the unwanted object of someone's attentions still raw, I felt instantly uneasy about working with her. I needed a stalker on my caseload like I needed a dose of Ebola. How was I going to find the objectivity I needed to build a rapport with her? And yet, personal worries aside, the professional in me was also curious. My thinking had made a major shift away from the strict diagnostic labels by that stage, but erotomania is fairly unusual and I was keen to know what it meant for Maya.

The word erotomania sounds increasingly Victorian in today's parlance. But in fact the idea has existed in medical texts for many hundreds of years, with no precise definition. It went through various incarnations and modifications via a range of psychiatric luminaries (including Sigmund Freud, who suggested the term described a way of repressing homosexual urges). The problem it now describes was first declared a syndrome by a French psychotherapist – G G de Clérambault – after he counselled a female patient who stood outside Buckingham Palace for hours at a time, certain that King George was communicating his love for her by moving the curtains. In 1942, his seminal paper 'Les Psychoses Passionnelles' was published and the phenomenon became widely known as De Clérambault syndrome, until erotomania joined the fourth edition of the DSM as a form of delusional disorder and superseded it.

Erotomania is simply the illusion of love. It describes a false belief, held by a person, that their target – most often someone older who occupies a higher social status than them – is passionately and irrevocably in love with them, although the target in question has often had little or no contact with the person labouring under the delusion. The diagnosis is more commonly applied to women than men, although men can also find themselves besotted by an indifferent, if not completely oblivious, sweetheart.

Erotomania was also known in the early 19th century as Old Maid's Insanity, the lack of a husband being presumed so harrowing for any woman over a certain age that it would push her into a state of amorous hysteria (no one's sure who coined that phrase but it almost certainly wasn't an old maid). I have always enjoyed the irony of this particular name, given what we now know about how men tend to struggle more with bachelorhood in old age – dying younger and developing more degenerative diseases such as dementia.

Once a person diagnosed with erotomania has 'established' their belief in the other person's desire for them, he or she will usually begin to reciprocate the imagined love. This could mean anything from leaving flowers on the doorstep to more overt declarations, to which they hope the target will respond favourably.

More often than not, the person with erotomania finds their romantic overtures rejected, so they start to generate reasons that excuse or explain the rebuff and continue to allow them to believe their target really is in love with them. It is common for them to come to the conclusion that an external force, such as someone's spouse, is standing between them and a life of unbridled bliss.

I was once asked for help by a man who believed the object of his affection's husband was holding her captive and that she must therefore have so-called Stockholm syndrome (where a hostage develops a seemingly paradoxical emotional attachment to the kidnapper). This was the only possible reason he could find for her refusal to run away with him, and he asked me to put the official stamp of diagnosis on her. He also put Wild West-style 'WANTED' posters up around his village, appealing for information that would help lead to the arrest of her family for holding her captive. He later appeared in court wearing a sheriff's outfit, accompanied by a miniature Shetland pony (who did not make it past door security checks). I wasn't available to assist the sheriff at the time, but part of me wishes I had been.

*

Maya first started hanging around the GP's surgery as a teenager, sitting in the waiting room after school even though she didn't have an appointment. When she was 16 she began to write cards and letters to one of the GPs,

Dr King, expressing her undying love for him. It seemed harmless enough at first, but her devotion didn't stop at teenage infatuation, and she had begun to wait for him outside the surgery and even followed him home a number of times.

Maya's behaviour gradually escalated to the point where she began threatening to hurt herself and Dr King if he didn't return her affections. She warned she would slit her wrists if he couldn't be hers, she would lie down in the road and kill herself.

Then one afternoon she had waited outside his consulting room while he was seeing a patient and, when the door opened at the end of the appointment, pushed her way into the room and locked the door behind her, ensuring she was alone with the doctor. Dr King had reached directly for his desk phone and called through to reception, and fortunately a nurse was able to unlock the door from the outside, but there had been a tussle and raised voices as Maya had tried to block her. As Dr King tried to open the door, Maya pushed him onto the examination couch and tried to climb on top of him. She simply wanted to be close to him, she said. It all sounded clumsy and vaguely farcical, but if you're the person being climbed on against your will in a locked room, it's likely to be a while before you can see the funny side.

As psychotherapist Frank Tallis points out in his book *The Incurable Romantic: And Other Unsettling Revelations*, there is a certain unsavoury pleasure to be found in watching people make fools of themselves in the name of 'love'. But 'when we mock the lovelorn, we do so as hypocrites or automatons. Who hasn't acted foolishly – or at least conspicuously out of character – when in love?' Who indeed. But Maya's fixation went far beyond simply making a nuisance of herself. When she began to deliver handwritten threats to kill Dr King's wife and children to his home, she was arrested and taken into the care of psychiatric services. Maya had put him and his family through a terrifying ordeal.

*

For the next 20 years, Maya had lived in one secure hospital after another, residing in locked psychiatric wards, gradually moving from high to medium and eventually low-security settings.

The reports in her considerable file showed she hadn't given up on doctors. The reports nearly always mentioned a psychologist, a psychiatrist or maybe a nurse with whom she was beguiled, although she was fickle and her allegiances drifted from professional to professional. One report described her as 'willing to show up for therapy but non-committal when she does and maintains declarations of love'. It seemed she was keen to be in the same room as the string of psychologists who had been tasked with her treatment over the years, but once there she would say very little apart from telling them repeatedly that she loved them.

For nearly twenty years, Dr King had remained a more consistent passion – she had continued to write letters to him since the episode at the surgery, although of course they were never sent. The letters were kept in her file. Looking through them it was clear from the earlier notes that she was someone in a state of genuine agony, they were long and intense pages of handwriting, spelling out her suffering in exacting and tortured detail and her fury that she and the love of her life, her destiny no less, were being kept apart.

Reports from her earlier years in hospital detailed how she described the voice of Dr King telling her to kill his wife to clear the way for their love. She talked about taking him hostage at knifepoint, if that was what it would take for them to be together at last. In the depths of her despair, when she felt most hopeless or rejected, she starved herself, scratched deep lines across her face and pierced her body with whatever sharp object she could get her hands on.

I noted that as time passed and she moved to lower-security wards, the letters became less and less frequent. They became briefer, less poetic and harrowed. They unravelled into a thin string of repetitive notes, 'I want you to know that I love you. I would do anything for you.' The notes read like someone paying lip service to a relationship that has long since lost its spark, as if writing it had been a job on her to-do list that day. The letters eventually stopped and she hadn't written to Dr King for a number of years by the time I met her.

Now she was the same age as me – 40; when life begins, so the greetings cards say – and the hope was that this would be her last hospital placement before her transition into 'real' life.

Things were looking positive for Maya.

*

But when I met her, it quite quickly became clear that she wasn't so keen on building a life for herself outside the oasis of the hospital walls.

During her very first meeting with her care team (me, the psychiatrist, the occupational therapist and the nurse in charge that day), she sat down and informed us forthrightly that she was a hopeless case. 'I've done it all before,' she said. 'Nothing can make me better.'

This seemed like a defeatist way to start proceedings. I took in the sparky, bright-faced woman in front of me. Her impossibly white teeth looked too perfect to be real, and I realized they were false. The straight line of perfect dentures looked just slightly too big for her mouth, which added to the overall impact of her. She had on the chunky yellow jumper that she wore all the time, it swamped her frame, and she tucked her thick dark hair behind her ears with efficiency and purpose as she spoke, her fingernails each painted a different shade. She had intricate swirls of red henna dye on her hands. She was full of colour.

How would you know that you are 'better'? I asked. What would better look or feel like? She couldn't answer. She was dangerous, she informed us. She had De Clérambault syndrome and she was 'treatment resistant'. She had all the jargon, and I was struck by how certain she was of what she saw as her irreversible condition. It seemed she saw it as her identity now. This wasn't so much a level of self-awareness as an exercise in locking down the situation on her terms.

Plus, she still heard the voice of Dr King telling her to kill his wife, she said. 'So that we can be together, that's all he ever says.'

I asked if she found the voice upsetting, and she was very matter of fact as she replied, Yes, it was awful, all-consuming and excruciating. This could have been what's known as a 'blunted affect', the emotion-flattening result of long-term mental ill-health and, often, the medication prescribed as a result. She looked at me as she shrugged and I wondered if Maya was really in as difficult a place as she wanted us to believe.

After that meeting, we each received the same short note from Maya, written in an elegant looped script. She wanted us to know that we were 'perfect and God-like' to her. She loved us and she would do anything for us.

*

One of the many worthwhile aspects of working with patients in a small environment like this hospital was being able to practise a more free-flow kind of psychology. With such a small number of patients it was far less structured and procedure driven, unbound by the conventions and routines of more densely populated places I'd worked. Alleluia. I found myself with the time, resources and autonomy to practise psychology as I saw fit. I wasn't chained slavishly to any particular treatment style, manualized programme or group timetable. I could spend time with the women there based on what level of support they needed, rather than the preordained hour once a week, no more, no less. The therapy we practised was tailored to be meaningful for each individual. I believe that psychology should be embedded into day-to-day life, in everything that we do. So I kept an open-door policy and patients came to me when they were struggling, as did the staff. There was still an element of form filling and auditing of course, but it didn't overtake the care of the patients.

Although there was one person who didn't make use of my open door. Or in fact anything else on offer in the hospital. Maya turned down invitations to join the local Hearing Voices Group – a small support group that might have helped her manage what she said were Dr King's instructions to kill his wife. She often didn't show up for her scheduled one-to-one appointments with me. We had started trialling a new form of therapy for people who were distressed by voices and it was getting some great results. When I asked Maya if she wanted to try it, she said no – if she lost Dr King's voice she would miss it. I've heard this before from people who hear voices, but given what she had said previously about the distress it caused her it didn't seem to make any logical sense. There was no rhyme nor reason to it (and that part of it at least sounded the most like love to me).

Maya turned down all my invitations to work with me, remarking 'you are a psychologist so you are up here' – she pointed to the sky – 'and I am down there' – and she pointed to the floor. She once told me that she liked to think that I spent all my time studying books and probably didn't even need to sleep, and certainly didn't use the toilet. Maya wanted me to know that, although she didn't want to do any work with me, she loved me nonetheless. In fact, she repeatedly said she would do anything for the staff at the hospital, and yet she did her level best to avoid any kind of actual treatment. She would do anything for love, but she wouldn't do that.

I decided not to ask Maya to keep her appointments with me in the way the other patients did, but instead to 'bump into' her around the hospital. This wasn't difficult as the place was so small. I became a psychologist in stealth mode. My hope was that by doing away with the formal trappings of my role – the quiet room and the notepad, the open-yet-concerned gaze across a coffee table – she might begin to see me as a human being on her level, rather than revere me as a deity.

On one occasion I quite genuinely bumped into her as I was coming out of the toilet, and in a moment of flippancy I said, 'I'd give it a few minutes if I were you.' This is not a technique you will find in any psychology textbook, but I was rather pleased with my own maverick genius – I'd used the chance to show her that I was a mere mortal, with bodily functions, and bring myself down off the pedestal she had me on. If her nose wrinkled as her psychologist made a terrible toilet gag, that was exactly what I wanted. I was determined to break down this ideal of health professionals.

Most of the other patients would go out during the day on walks and trips, attending work and appointments alone or with staff, but Maya never wanted to go. She stayed in the communal lounge watching TV. There was always some American sitcom on. She liked the ones about families, with canned laughter and wisecracking kids. Sitcoms, schmaltzy made-for-TV films and anything with Tom Hanks in. She loved Tom Hanks. Kind, non-threatening, smiley-faced Tom Hanks.

One morning I found her in the communal lounge, where she was again watching TV. She wasn't expecting me, and I sat down beside her, and we both half-watched the programme and half-talked. A big St Bernard dog came on in the show she was watching and she said she loved dogs so I showed her a picture of my two. This is what's called 'appropriate self-disclosure'. Psychologists don't, as a rule, share personal information with patients, but if it is safe and you think it will be helpful, sharing a little part of yourself can be a useful tool. I never tell anyone anything about my family or relationships, and with Maya's history in particular I wouldn't let any personal details of that nature slip. But I had discovered that my dogs were a safe go-to subject, the perfect leveller. Who doesn't love dogs after all? I showed Maya one of Fozzchops where she had got a cream cheese triangle stuck to her ear and she really laughed at it – lost herself for a few seconds and just snorted with glee. A small glimpse into my perfectly imperfect life.

We sat and chatted like this whenever the opportunity presented itself. I started to understand her in those moments. Slowly we were lifting the veil of her diagnosis to see what lay beneath it. Those chats with Maya remain among some of my favourite experiences as a psychologist, building trust, doing it the way I felt it should be done, one old maid to another.

With no pressure from me she began to confide in me more and more. She was revealing herself in many ways, not least as being good company. Just as she was beginning to engage with me, I was also warming to her. The stalker I had feared I would struggle to work with was turning out to be quite funny and smart. She told me once that she liked Dr King's eyes. When I asked why, she said he had 'footballer's eyes'. I said I didn't understand what she meant and she replied, well, they pointed in different directions, one was 'playing at home and the other was playing away'. I never pushed her on the subject of Dr King but I did enjoy this description of him. We used to make up funny book titles together: *Back Problems* by Eileen Bent or *The Art of Bull Fighting* by Matt Adore. She had heard Terry Wogan on the radio in the morning doing something similar and she loved the silliness. In between she talked to me about her past and her family, and told me all about her dad. I found that I liked her. She was bright and had a lot to offer the world.

The time I spent with her also helped me soften mildly – and only mildly – towards the man who had stalked me. I was finding my balance again. The patient– therapist relationship is a two-way street. The benefits to the psychologist of a therapeutic alliance are rarely discussed, but they do occasionally happen.

But all the feelings of hope and optimism I had about Maya's recovery were most often quashed. She stalled. She didn't want to leave the hospital alone or even go on any of the accompanied outings with the hospital staff that the other patients did. Just at the point when I felt she might take tentative steps into the outside world and begin to imagine a new life for herself, at the hint of an excursion into reality she would always pull back. And always the same response: No, no, I am ill, I am sick. And if we pushed her: No. I am dangerous. Dr King is telling me to kill his wife. On one or two occasions she scratched herself, and once drew a shallow but decisive line onto her face with a CD.

One day I asked Maya to describe to me her idea of a perfect place, somewhere she would go if she couldn't be here. She told me it would be a long hospital corridor, entirely bare but with doors leading off it on either side. She could walk up and down this corridor and open any door she liked, and inside every room would be a doctor who she could stay with for as long as she wanted to. They would make sure that she was fed and taken care of. At night, they would tuck her into bed.

This sorry vision of a hospital-based utopia made me think of my Uncle John's canary, who had spent a lifetime in a cage and preferred to stay there, even when the doors were open.

I'd witnessed something similar a few years before, when visiting a medium-secure unit in the north-east to give evidence at a Mental Health Review Tribunal. It was a grand old sanatorium-style place, shiny pale bricks and long, tall windows, with a winding tree-lined drive that felt like a portal into a Brontë novel.

I had been asked to wait in one of the admin offices with the mental health administrator and two secretaries. The room had a window overlooking an ugly gravelled courtyard with a smoking area and a set of huge iron gates.

As we waited, the pale grey sky in the window turned all of a sudden to a menacing shade of ash and there was a huge crack of thunder. An enormous storm was coming in. We all gathered around the window to watch the blackening sky and saw that, below us, a few patients were huddled together in the smoking area like penguins, sucking rapidly on their cigarettes, their hands cupped around them, trying to keep them dry.

Then there was another almighty crack and instinctively we all looked up to the sky, expecting to see lightning. But there was no lightning and we realized the noise had been the wind blowing one of the big iron gates into the courtyard with such force that it had snapped the chain lock and come loose from the other gate. Suddenly the gates were open and the smokers beneath us were only a few feet away from a tantalizingly easy exit.

One of the patients ran towards it – he was skinny and tall, with a long stride. I couldn't see his face from where I was, but he was wearing a blue woolly bobble hat, and I watched as the hat travelled at speed towards the entrance, expecting to see him zoom out into the middle distance. But he stopped just short of the gates. He took a couple of steps backwards and one tentative step forward, flapping his arms around indecisively. Just like Uncle John's canary.

The other patients had all run inside and a nurse was

standing at the doorway calling the potential escapee to come back in. He stood looking at the gates for a few more seconds, the heavens now fully opened above him, then he turned around and scurried inside.

As the patients trooped past the office we were waiting in, we made the obligatory comments about the Armageddon-like squall outside. The man in the hat was soaked through to the skin.

'Look at me! It's raining bloody cats and bloody dogs out there.' He stretched his arms out. 'I'm not running off. Not today, not in that weather.'

I shook my head and said, 'Nooo, you'll catch your death in this!'

'I know,' he said. 'I'd rather stay here. It's a shithole but at least I can get a decent brew.'

How very British, I thought to myself.

*

A locum psychiatrist came to work at the hospital for a week, and before Maya had even met him she sent him a love note, declaring, 'I love you I would do anything for you.' Unlike the rest of us, he was furious about this note. He considered it a boundary violation and sent it back to her with a clear message that he would not accept it.

Maya came to my office – at last – and threw herself down in the chair. She said, 'But he is my doctor, it is his job to take care of me.' There was that sense of entitlement written in the sulk on her face.

I explained that yes it was his job to take care of safely prescribing her medication, but that it was just that, a job, and he was clearly very personally offended by her note. She thought about it for a moment and declared, 'Being sick makes you selfish.'

Was it being sick? Or just wanting to feel safe? I asked her this because I understood that, to some extent, I was working at that hospital seeking the same thing – a sense of security, a safe harbour. I told her that wanting to feel safe was completely understandable. In fact, I believed that she was entitled to that, but not at the expense of someone else feeling unsafe.

She nodded slightly and then said, 'I do love doctors, but I would probably run a mile if one ever wanted me. A doctor would never look at me. They are too good for me. I just want them to take care of me.'

After Maya left my office that day, she didn't cut herself, threaten anybody or mention Dr King again. I was certain then that Maya was better and had been for some time. The all-consuming illusion of love had long-since dissipated to nothing more than a pleasant fantasy to call upon, and a mantra to ensure she remained cared for.

*

Doctors had come to represent much more to Maya than mere healers. In that simple act of tucking her into bed, the doctor who had visited her years ago had given her a glimpse of the love and care she had never received from her father. Dr King had rejected her romantic advances but had rescued her nonetheless: her infatuation with him had led to her detention, removing her from the danger of her family home. And now, with a lifetime spent in institutions behind her, the idea of taking responsibility for herself, leaving the safety and security of the hospital and the doctors was terrifying. Infinitely more terrifying, even, than remaining 'sick'.

Long after her abusive childhood, a basic need to feel safe drove Maya to maintain her 'sick' identity. Like the bobble-hatted man, Maya took tentative steps towards her freedom; coming to see and accept me as human like her had been a huge step forward. And yet she wasn't quite ready to make it past the gates either, finding reasons to stay in the safety of the hospital and rejecting the help that might propel her outwards into the world. This is the nature of therapy sometimes – one step forward, one step back. You keep on going all the same.

The allure and sanctity of the 'sick role', as it is known in psychology, is complex. Mental health professionals have long recognized that there are those in the system for whom the idea of being a patient beats the idea of not. I have seen similar in prison environments too.

To those of us for whom freedom is a given it seems unbelievable that someone wouldn't want that liberty for themselves. But what is privacy and independence for some can feel like isolation and insecurity for others. When life in the outside world is an unkind and uncertain prospect, the psychiatric set up offers care and sanctuary. And as unlikely a settling-down territory as it may seem, stay somewhere long enough and it can become a home, even a family.

In order for someone to feel strong enough to move on, they need to be able to picture a better life for themselves, one that is achievable, that is better than the one they're living. As their therapeutic ally, the psychologist can only really show them what that life might look like. You shine the light, and hobble with them to the end of the tunnel, but you can't make them step out. For some the light is blinding.

CHAPTER 11
THE SUM OF OUR PARTS

The whole is greater than the sum of its parts.
Aristotle

Before its incarnation as a women's psychiatric hospital, the stuccoed Victorian villa where I worked with Jeane had been a bed and breakfast. From time to time people would still walk down the long tree-lined drive to knock at the door, asking if we had any vacancies. I loved imagining what the TripAdvisor reviews might have said if we'd have welcomed them in.

It was part of the same group of small and friendly recovery centres for women where I had worked with Maya, and I had been with them for some time now. Like the others in the group, it felt more like a home than a hospital. It had old-fashioned Anaglypta wallpaper obscured under layers of old paint, shaggy carpets and dark, musty-smelling floral curtains. *World of Interiors* it wasn't, but it helped the residents feel at ease, like living on the inside of a giant knitted tea cosy. Although this exercise in faded grandeur was less pleasant for us staff: the ancient heating system in my office meant that if it wasn't fridge-like it was tropical, a situation made worse by the fact I couldn't keep the door open because of fire regulations, or open the window because, like all the windows, there was a bar across it.

There were nine bedrooms here, with the residents ranging in age from nineteen through to sixty. They were all women with complex mental health struggles. It was a diverse group, including women who heard threatening voices, had memory problems caused by addiction, or who'd had high-flying careers until the compulsion to wash or pick at their skin had overwhelmed them. I liked that we appeared to have no rigid admissions criteria; no typical story bound these women, other than our shared belief that we could help them. There was a lot of warmth and compassion in the place. In fact, of all the hospitals I've worked in, it remains up there in terms of its aspirations and the standard of genuine care it gave. But I came to realize that even in a homely, caring environment like this, compassion comes with conditions and caveats.

Jeane was referred to us after being found by police when she was about to throw herself off a motorway bridge. She'd been taken to the acute ward of an NHS hospital and I'd been asked to assess her suitability for a place with us. It turned out Jeane had been trying to kill herself one way or another for a few weeks; the reports said 'ligatured' (when someone tries to hang or strangle themselves) and gave a series of dates on which she had tried to cause herself harm. On one occasion she'd tied herself to the back of her wardrobe door with a blanket and they'd found her unconscious. Another time, she'd tried to cut her wrists with the jagged edges of a Coke can. In her arm she'd scratched the word 'bad' with a piece of glass. She was sending some very clear signals that she needed help.

Jeane's paperwork revealed she'd spent much of her late teens and early adulthood in and out of psychiatric care. But she had also spent long periods of time living an outwardly unremarkable life – long enough to get married and raise two children. She was in her 40s now, but when she'd discovered her husband was having an affair, and he'd cruelly asked her to leave so he could move his mistress in, she had started to flounder.

The first thing I noticed about Jeane was her other-worldly aura; she often looked as if she were drifting, like she had swallowed a big cloud. The effect was made all the more incongruous by her hulking size and build. She was five feet ten, and almost as wide; silver haired, with a ruddy complexion, she looked like she could single-handedly plough a field. Intently squeezing a string of blue beads as she spoke in her slow, light and delicate voice, she explained that she was desperate to understand what was happening to her, and to break out of the pattern of self-destruction she found herself in. She was reaching out for an escape from her situation; from all the confusion and guilt she was feeling and her fear of what might happen next. I felt certain that we could work with Jeane to turn things around.

My enthusiasm in wanting to bring Jeane into our eclectic group wasn't shared by my colleagues, however. Jeane had been given a diagnostic label that can be interpreted in many different, and often pejorative, ways by mental health staff: 'borderline personality disorder' (BPD, also sometimes referred to as 'emotionally unstable personality disorder').

For starters, the criteria used to diagnose BPD feel more like a rap sheet than a set of symptoms or difficulties: self-harming and all-round reckless behaviour (unsafe sex, outbursts of rage, drug use and so on) are the big markers, along with violent mood swings and a paranoid mistrust of others. Meanwhile, the characteristics and personality traits associated with a BPD label can read like the definitive list of all the reasons ever invented not to like someone. Such people can be irritable, self-destructive, clingy, wildly unpredictable and generally quite annoying for everyone around them. There's an unhelpful tendency, even among those caring for them, to see this disproportionately female group as manipulative and attention-seeking. The term 'drama queen' was probably coined – unfairly – about someone tagged with BPD.

What's certain is that whatever a person with this label is doing, they aren't having a good time, or trying to provoke people merely for the hell of it. Yet the term 'personality disorder' is innately accusatory; the diagnostic equivalent of a wagging finger. These people have been bruised; describing them as disordered makes it sound like their character, their innermost core, is somehow wilfully and irretrievably flawed.

When a few days later Jeane arrived to check in at the hospital, I noticed there was something different about her. She was, expectedly, anxious. But she was also uncommunicative with the staff, and when she did speak her voice was even higher-pitched, more nasal and childlike. It didn't help that she was dressed in pink jeans and a pink top with a pony on it – the kind of outfit a nine-year-old girl might pick out. She planted herself on the sofa in the hospital lounge surrounded by a menagerie of cuddly toys she had brought with her. One of these, a huge cat, became as much a resident of the place as Jeane. It had a patch over one eye and mismatched ears, the kind of loveable stray you see in children's books. We had to restuff it at one point, because it had nearly been cuddled into extinction.

I clocked a couple of the usually kind-hearted nurses roll their eyes at each other when she arrived, as if to say,

Here we go. Even before she had had any professional attention, Jeane's copybook already had a big fat BPD-shaped blot on it. Beneath the gaze of even these dedicated nurses, she had been labelled as difficult, possibly beyond help, before she had barely got through the door.

That wasn't the only reason for my unease. As soon as I had encountered this floating woman in the acute ward of the hospital, I felt that her predicament didn't even correspond to the already broad and unhelpfully loaded category of BPD. If we had to slap a label on Jeane, it should at least offer a more accurate description of her issues. Her difficulties were more consistent with what is known as 'dissociative identity disorder' (DID).

Previously known as having multiple personalities, people attracting the DID diagnosis in fact have only one personality, but they experience it as distinct and separate parts. The switch between the different parts of their personality can be very subtle, as simple as a change in mannerisms or tone of voice. Or it can be more obvious: someone can feel physically different, a different gender even, or reveal skills or habits their 'regular' self doesn't seem to share. They can also be entirely unaware of the switch, and experience a kind of amnesia when it happens, travelling to different places and not remembering how they got there. Jeane's reports showed she did this frequently; she had been picked up in random places on the other side of town, clueless as to how she'd arrived. Understandably, the accompanying lack of control and sense of powerlessness was terrifying, adding another thread to the already complex knot of emotional trauma involved. Most importantly, the symptoms aligned with DID are a consequence of severe physical and sexual abuse in childhood – something I would learn Jeane had endured on an immense scale as a little girl.

As a child, she had learned to cope with the abject horror of her childhood abuse by cutting off from and 'floating' outside herself. Her memories of that time had become fragmented, and emerged – usually uninvited – in the form of these alter egos. Hence the pink outfits and the cuddly toys – they were physical props, the cherished possessions of her alternative selves. These personalities were the manifestations of her recollections and emotions stuck in time, ring-fenced and given names of their own.

*

We began twice-weekly therapy sessions and normally she gave it her all. I wanted to help her understand her distress in the context of what had happened to her, and to make her self-harming less frequent and, more importantly, less likely to be lethal. Between us, we started to piece together her story.

Most often she talked to me as Jeane, and other times she talked to me as one of her alters. She experienced intensely physical flashbacks; sometimes she would choke and even vomit. The sex offenders I'd worked with tended not to mention certain details, like how their victim threw up during the abuse or how they had gagged so much that they couldn't breathe. It's only when you work directly with victims that the full, unsanitized horror of abuse becomes clear.

Jeane hadn't told anyone the candid story of her life and it felt like an enormous privilege to be entrusted with it, to be a witness for her and to guide her gently back to the here and now when a flashback engulfed her. I wanted to help her understand that what was happening to her was an understandable response to what she had been through, and to reassure the different parts of herself that she wasn't in danger any more.

Jeane was the only patient who I've ever allowed to see me cry. For an unsentimental and usually hard-nosed forensic psychologist tears in front of a client would usually be a big no-no, but I felt it was unavoidable with Jeane. After all, it was my genuine, human response to her story. She needed to know that what had happened to her was wrong and someone was genuinely sorry that it was allowed to happen.

Ten-year-old Claire was the most frequent of Jeane's identities to appear. Claire co-existed with her, and acted as her trusted helper and friend. Claire told me how her earliest memories were of watching her brother being abused by her father and his friends. Over the course of our time together, it became apparent that Jeane's father had been part of an organized paedophile ring, who Jeane and her brother had been trafficked by.

If Claire was Jeane's ally, someone she could call when she felt scared, her other alter Drew was the troublemaker. It was Drew who drove much of Jeane's destructive behaviour, the suicide attempts and the self-harming. It was Drew who was often the most difficult part of Jeane for the hospital staff to accept.

Interestingly, Drew was also the name of Jeane's older brother. At 16 he had run away from home and she never saw him again. He had gone on to take his own life, something Jeane only heard about years later. The thought that her brother had died and then been buried alone was unbearable for Jeane. Drew then was the part of her who carried the most intense loss, anger and guilt she felt about her brother. After dissociating into Drew, when she was consciously Jeane again, she would deny all knowledge of Drew's behaviour. To the staff at the hospital, already sceptical, this seemed like an all-too-convenient and suspicious loss of memory. They found Drew's antics unacceptable.

Jeane's third alter, Belle, didn't speak at all. Perhaps she was trapped in a time when she was too young for speech, or maybe there just weren't the words. But she drew pictures.

Faceless men holding children's hands. Belle was left-handed, while Jeane was right-handed. I sometimes sat and watched as Belle quietly drew with her left hand while Jeane wrote with her right, both hands working at the same time. It was, admittedly, an eerie thing to see. Staff began to whisper that Jeane seemed possessed.

It struck me, not for the first (or last) time, that here were otherwise highly competent mental health professionals who were more comfortable talking in terms of demonic possession, or insisting their patient was a devious manipulator, than accepting the logical, psychological formulation of Jeane's behaviour: that she had broken her sense of self down into disparate parts in what was an elaborate and creative survival strategy. Jeane was not possessed. Just divided. That, and ambidextrous.

But maybe, in their own way, the staff were also dissociating. Perhaps their empathy and disgust for what Jeane had been put through was too much for them to make sense of. Or maybe the reality of Jeane's experience and of those like her is too alien for anyone from the comfort of a relatively normal background to fully comprehend. But I was unfortunate enough to have been a witness to the murky world of paedophilia through my work with offenders, and understood what she had been through without the need for much imagination. Perhaps I was more able to accept what had happened to her. Jeane's 'disorder' had in fact been an effective and essential strategy for her during the years she was being abused, but dissociating was far less helpful to her in adulthood. Having used this strategy for practically her whole life, I knew it was unlikely she was going to be able to stop altogether – to be able to fully accept all her thoughts, feelings, experiences and memories as her own and become a single 'I' rather than a multiple 'we'. (Although, if we are honest, do any of us really fully embrace every aspect of ourselves?) Besides, giving up Claire, who she thought of as a reassuring friend, would have been a grave loss to her. So through our sessions we worked towards a point where she wasn't putting herself in danger any more, where if she felt she was drifting off into unsafe corners of her mind – into Drew – she could pull herself back with simple grounding techniques. This could be something as easy as making herself aware of her feet on the ground or using her worry beads to bring her awareness back to her body, focusing on objects in her environment and naming them out loud.

On the anniversary of her brother's death we planted an apple tree for him in the grounds of the hospital and talked about, and celebrated, his life. By these small acts of validation, we were taking steps towards healing her trauma.

*

Therapeutically, I felt our sessions were a success. But outside of the psychology sessions, things weren't so rosy. Jeane wasn't toeing the line. As a hospital resident she was expected to get up by a certain time, eat the meals provided at the set time, take part in a scheduled programme of activities, be observed bathing and – most difficult for Jeane – drop her trousers at the required time to be injected with medication.

This wasn't in a prison or a secure hospital, Jeane didn't have any forensic history or criminal convictions, and yet here again were the ways in which institutions insist upon taking away autonomy and dignity, controlling the individual.

Jeane didn't like it, and she made it clear when she didn't want to follow the rules. She got embroiled in disputes with staff about petty issues. One morning there was a screaming match because she hadn't been allowed to eat crisps for breakfast. We wanted her to behave more consistently as an adult, and yet she wasn't granted the freedom to make an adult decision for herself. She shouted, slammed doors, stomped about and threw things, all in front of the other patients.

As her psychologist, I felt torn. Jeane was being vilified for her unruly behaviour (one nurse said, 'I'm here to help people who are poorly, she's just being naughty'). But I couldn't help privately admiring her fight, and feeling proud that she still had the spirit in her to say no. Being robbed of her right to say no as a child was what brought her here in the first place.

I say, let her tell a few people to fuck off if she wants to. Can't we – the lucky ones – be more respectful of the way the victims of abuse respond to their trauma, instead of ladling on extra shame and guilt when they don't eat the breakfast we want them to? Why do we find it so difficult to appreciate that the experiences of abused children, often by the people they trust most, are among the most harmful things a human being can ever endure? And what are we aiming for in rehabilitating a person anyway? Someone who is passively compliant or someone with a sense of their own agency?

Jeane was the subject of some particularly unpleasant debates in our team meetings at the hospital. The manager wanted us to clamp down on her, and even suggested we could show her who was in charge by restraining her next time she became argumentative.

Physically holding her down, like something from a *Panorama* exposé, would have not only been unnecessary but deeply retraumatizing, as it would have so closely mirrored her abuse. The dark art of teaching someone a lesson isn't part of any good psychologist's toolkit, and restraint-as-punishment was simply never going to happen on my watch – Jeane was obnoxious and insulting, and her size was intimidating, but she was never a true physical threat. That particular meeting ended with the hospital manager walking out of the room (lucky, as I was going to need restraining myself had it gone on any longer). It occurred to me that despite the cheerful diversity of our residents, there was, after all, an unwritten admission criterion here, a subtle cherry-picking of patients who wouldn't be 'difficult'.

All the heat around Jeane was propelling her further and faster to the inevitable conclusion. For hospital staff, it was just more evidence of her BPD. Hadn't they known it from the start? The more Jeane resisted the rules and expectations of the hospital, the more rules and expectations were heaped on her; the staff's distaste for her became palpable, especially to her, feeding her own deep sense of being inherently bad. A self-fulfilling prophecy was playing out.

Then one day Jeane broke a window and went AWOL. Police found her drinking Bacardi Breezers in the park. She said Drew did it (the window bit anyway, the drinking was unashamedly Jeane) but the nursing staff didn't believe her. I did though, and I explained to her again that Drew was the angry part of herself, and that Jeane had to take responsibility for it, which she accepted. But despite her willingness to learn in therapy, she wasn't able to comply in the way the institution wanted her to within the timeframe it wanted this to happen.

I eventually had to concede that our tea-cosy hospital wasn't the right place for her, although I will never concede it was her fault. Too often we deem patients unsuitable for care, when we should be trying harder to provide care that's more suitable for them.

On the day she left, she was picked up by the staff from the supported bedsit she'd been allocated, where she would get the help of a care worker six hours a week. Before she went, she tore the apple tree she'd planted for her brother straight out of the ground. She left crying, begging to be allowed to stay, promising she'd be good and not misbehave again, pleas all made in the language of a repentant child, still clutching her stuffed toy cat.

I often wonder how Jeane got on. She once sent me a Facebook friend request, which as her former therapist I couldn't accept. I hope she continued with therapy though.

She always thought what had happened to her was somehow her fault. She especially blamed herself for her brother's suicide. I hope she realized it wasn't.

*

That was summer 2016 – I didn't know it then but by October that year I would have quit my job at the women's hospital. I had genuinely loved working there, helping women pick up the reins of their lives and waving them off to new beginnings. In truth most of them were champing at the bit to resume their freedom, while other more reluctant leavers (like 'love-sick' Maya, who did eventually move on to a more independent home) went with what one of my favourite nurses referred to as 'Ugg therapy' – the softest of kicks up the backside to help them on the way. Being part of that group of small hospitals, where the care was individualized and meaningful, was as close as I had come to practising the kind of psychology I felt had most impact.

But Jeane had left us, not quite kicking and screaming, but still in real distress, begging to be allowed to stay. She wanted to work through her trauma, and we had denied her safe passage. That ruthless moment had left a bitter taste in my mouth, and no amount of rinsing and spitting could seem to get rid of it. I'd dedicated myself to working with women with only the most optimistic of mindsets, but had discovered that the system didn't work for victims like Jeane any more than it did for offenders. The indignation I felt after watching Mark Bridger's trial was still there, it had just relocated, an ache that had moved from one limb to another.

Then, shortly after her departure, a series of events made me wonder if I was in fact colluding with something bigger, feeding a monster who had been hiding in plain sight all along.

Jeane left on Friday and on the next Sunday morning I was almost run over by a car outside my house. I was taking one of my dogs out, enjoying the simple feeling of sunshine on my face. The car – a bland, middle-management kind of model – came up out of nowhere, swerved quickly into me and out again, narrowly missing mounting the kerb and knocking me or Fozzchops over. No one was hurt, but it seemed like a very deliberate attempt to make me feel momentarily in peril. The road was quiet and empty – there had been no other reason to lurch my way.

Then the car slowed to a crawl next to me, and the man inside looked directly at me and laughed. I was in the midst of making some very unseemly hand gestures when it came to me. Was it him? It looked like him, but I couldn't tell. I had deliberately avoided looking him in the face in court, and besides I hadn't heard from him since 2012. But something about that moment and the way the car stopped for those few seconds made me feel this was no accident.

Then a week later I got his bill. The same man who had built those unsolicited websites now said I owed him £26,000 and he would be taking me to a business court for non-payment. He included an itemized bill, with a full breakdown of the costs I had apparently incurred, including time he had spent on researching me, the money he had spent on property searches and – what made me really laugh out loud – £500 on travel expenses.

His letter included an invitation to negotiate. He was willing to meet with me, he said, and thrash this out in a 'round table' meeting, as if he was a prime minister extending me a diplomatic invite and not the man who had made my life a misery. I laughed again because the audacity was fleetingly very funny. And then it wasn't.

Once again, I had to hire a solicitor to deal with his nonsense, who wrote to him explaining that I would not be attending his round table gathering, however good the biscuits were. The case was thrown out as an abuse of court process, just as I knew it would be. But I found myself thinking – this really was an inconceivable state of affairs, in which a total stranger could intimidate and then invoice me, simply, it seemed, for being alive. I had altered the way I worked, avoided appearing in public, kept my head down trying not to attract any attention, and still he billed me for the pleasure. It dawned on me that I was all but colluding in the dynamics of an abusive relationship.

And then my cat Bijou died.

I had let the dogs out into the garden one morning and Bijou slunk out along with them. I popped upstairs to have a shower and get dressed, and came back down to let the dogs in for their breakfast. It was a routine we had going and we all knew the drill. Only this morning was different. When I opened the back door again the dogs wouldn't come back in. Instead they were sat staring at something at the foot of the side fence.

It was Bijou's fluffy body, lying limp and inert. I ran to him and knew immediately that he was dead; there was no movement and no sound. His mouth was pulled back so you could see white gums and his teeth. My instant response was to turn to Fozzchops, who was sitting there shifting her gaze between me and the now departed Bijou, and ask her quite sternly whether she had done this. I don't know what kind of answer I was expecting from a chow-chow, who looked as puzzled as I was, but that's what I did.

Deep down I knew that this wasn't the work of another animal. Years of looking at crime scene pictures helped me reach some swift conclusions. There wasn't a mark on Bijou's body, no blood, no sign of a tussle and no teeth had been sunk into him. And besides, I knew he could outrun both of the dogs if he needed to. As I looked closer, I could see that his body was in an unnatural position. He had his front legs underneath him and his head turned to the side, as if he had been thrown over the fence already dead. Had someone run him over and slung him into the garden? Or had someone twisted his neck? I couldn't say. Bijou was my dear companion for 16 years and I would never know how he died.

One thing I could say with certainty, though, was that Bijou hadn't been the one who picked up the pen and wrote 'JILL DANDO' on the fence. (Had my cat chosen to pick up a Bic and write his own epitaph at that moment it would almost certainly have said something like 'Goodbye and thanks for all the Dreamies', his favourite snack.) I didn't even see it until the next day when I went to put the bin out, with the remains of Bijou's last meal among the waste. It wasn't even written in big letters, no sinister red paint dripping down the slats like you'd get in a bad horror film. Just a plain-looking scrawl in biro on the outward facing side of the fence, as if a kid had been dared to do it by his friends, but had bottled it at the last minute and done it quickly, hoping no one would see.

Jill Dando. The journalist and *Crimewatch* presenter who was fatally shot outside her home in 1999 and whose killer has never been found. Five years ago my stalker had told readers of his website to 'stay tuned… watch this space'. Was this the threat of violence I had been waiting for?

Police arrested him and gave him a Harassment Warning for sending me the letters demanding settlement of his bill. This is a way of making it clear to someone that their act has caused harassment and if there are further allegations then the police can make an arrest. It struck me as an entirely inappropriate response to a behaviour defined by obsession and fixation. Handing him yet another bit of paper with my name on to add to his collection, fuelling his unfounded sense of having some sort of relationship or connection to me. It seemed to add insult to psychological injury.

I felt the anger rise again. Only this time it wasn't so visceral or unwieldy. It was more determined. Receiving that invoice from a man I had never met, a man who had verbally abused and defamed me and made me feel threatened in my own home, helped crystallize my thinking. It was suddenly very clear that no amount of keeping my head down was going to make a difference.

Filing my paperwork – a second set of court documents – in my now bulging file on this irritating and uninvited situation, I thought of Jeane, and the way we had labelled and then rejected her, pathologized and retraumatized her, even though she hadn't even committed a crime. And suddenly every single part of the system seemed broken to me. At each and every point on the matrix – criminals and victims, rich and poor, men and women, black and white – there were glaring inequalities and failures wherever you looked. Systemic failures at every level, from the moment a crime is or isn't reported to the solutions on offer. And I had to ask myself again, had I been part of the problem all along? I had been working within the criminal justice system for all these years, trying to muddle my way through the maze and get the best outcomes possible for my clients, and the public. But was I propping up a system that worked for a select few but failed everybody else?

I thought of Jeane pulling that tree out of the ground, roots and all, and hurling it across the lawn. She had gone out fighting and I knew I needed to harness her spirit. She didn't have the voice or the privilege or the platform that I had – but I could do something for her, if I used the insight she had given me.

I knew I could make a difference, but only by ripping my own roots out of the ground, making myself part of the solution rather than part of the problem. My stalker liked to invite me to 'watch this space', the unspecified promise of something unclear and yet entirely sinister. But as my mum would say, 'Knickers to that.' I had spent too long with my head down, watching this space. It was time for me to fill the space instead.

EPILOGUE

I'm still a forensic psychologist, but these days I choose to effect change by other routes. Part of my day job still involves acting as an expert witness in court and, even after all these years, I'm still never quite sure what each week will bring. But I have also harnessed my inner activist and become a campaigner for change on the issues that really matter to me. Rather than feeling compromised and frustrated within the system, I am trying to effect change from the outside.

I serve as a proud patron of the National Centre for Domestic Violence, and have been working to support a number of other charities, including the Suzy Lamplugh Trust. This organization works to reduce the risk of violence and aggression through campaigning, education and advocacy for victims. The charity was set up in memory of Suzy Lamplugh who disappeared in 1986 during the course of her work as an estate agent while showing a client round a house. In 2017, I started training police on improving the way they respond to reports of stalking behaviour, which after my own experience I knew was largely inadequate. This wasn't because police officers didn't care. The training and guidance on dealing with stalking was almost non-existent, despite a number of high-profile murders. In 2018, the Crown Prosecution Service and National Police Chiefs' Council announced a new joint package of improvement measures. These included clear instruction that Harassment Warnings should not be used in stalking cases, as they fail to address the root of the stalker's obsession, and the introduction of new procedures that ensure that risky patterns of behaviour are identified swiftly by police.

The campaign for a dedicated stalking protection bill continued into 2019. We asked for the introduction of Stalking Protection Orders, which would give police the authority to enforce early measures to immediately protect victims, and to ensure that stalkers get the psychological treatment they need to prevent further offending. This was passed into law in March 2019, and there is still much work to be done to ensure it works in practice.

I'm fortunate to have a media platform from which to raise awareness of these issues. Through the media I am trying to promote better conversations around both crime and mental distress. I'm firmly of the mind that the well-worn crime and mental 'illness' narratives we absorb via the media largely serve only to perpetuate stereotypes, stigmatize and stoke the kind of black-and-white thinking that gets everyone precisely nowhere. The more nuanced and measured we can be in our reporting of crime, the better our conversations around how to tackle crime will be. We need news reports and television programmes that are brave enough to ask the difficult questions so that we can start to look for more effective solutions.

When I was a year into my first university degree in 1993, then Prime Minister John Major urged us all to 'condemn a little more and understand a little less'. Since then, whichever political party has been in charge, understanding seems to have been abandoned altogether.

Condemnation is a message which speaks to a human instinct: the desire to distance ourselves as far and as fast as we can from the people and ideas that threaten us. When we are faced with crimes and the people who commit them, it is far easier to shout, 'Throw away the key!' and then look away – out of sight, out of mind – than try to get to the underlying causes. Criminal behaviours challenge us – and I should know because I have been personally and professionally challenged. I haven't always found it easy. Far from it. There have been times when I've felt extremes of both empathy and anger. We cannot allow either emotion to set the tone for how we respond to those who have committed crimes or who are in an extreme state of distress. I know that the balance between cool, objective reasoning with respect for the rights of others – what Paul Bloom refers to in his book *Against Empathy* as 'rational compassion' – is difficult to achieve. But achieve it we must.

I've come to realize that whenever I am asked 'What is wrong with these people?' it has really been an exercise in 'othering' my clients. We categorize rule-breakers as 'mad' or 'bad' – they must be one or the other – we say they did this because they were psychopathic, evil or [insert Disorder Of The Day]. For some of 'these people' it provides a convenient label to hide behind. It demonizes others and can make even themselves wonder if they are beyond redemption.

If your reaction to that is a shrug of your shoulders, I understand. But consider that not only do we 'other' criminals, we do the same to victims too. Too often we hear that a person was targeted because they were naive, vulnerable, promiscuous or put themselves in harm's way. Then we pathologize their distressed reactions to being victimized. The label of dysfunction we tar them with can almost entirely dictate their experience in the years ahead.

Yet where is it getting us? Our criminal justice system is not fit for purpose. The attitude towards offenders of 'They are sick in the head; they're not like us' mirrors the exact sentiment that has left the criminal justice system – from police shortages, to disappearing Legal

Aid, through to prisons – in its present precarious state.

The system we use to 'correct' extreme behaviours too often traumatizes and/or retraumatizes, institutionalizes and marginalizes those it aims to fix. Our prisons in particular provide the perfect conditions for the flourishing of the very problems we hope to eliminate.

Deep-rooted, far-reaching changes are needed, not political slogans and repeat prescriptions. It starts with an acknowledgement that, ultimately, we are all in this together. It is time to change the question, from 'What is wrong with them?' to altogether more awkward, uncomfortable questions. Let's start with: What has happened to them? And what has happened to us as a society?

These questions are fundamental, because while we continue to use explanations that situate the causes of extreme behaviour inside an individual – be it the perpetrator or, worse, the victim – we overlook the external forces. Factors that influence people's behaviour: our laws, culture, the gender expectations that are heaped on us from birth, and the media influences that foster violence and abuse in our society. We need to consider extremes of behaviour in their wider context: experiences of abuse and adversity; societal issues such as racism and other forms of discrimination; political and economic factors; exclusion, disenfranchisement and disempowerment.

One of my former clients, a Freddie Mercury lookalike, once watched an almighty argument between two of my colleagues. The pair had squared up to each other during an anger management group. One had punched the other in the face, giving him a bloody nose, much to the amusement of their patients, who clapped and cheered ringside. My client thought about this incident regularly and would tell me that it led him to the firm conclusion that 'psychologists are human too'.

We all share one fundamental condition – being human. And one of the things that makes us distinctly human is our capacity to choose to rise above our emotions when we need to, and in doing so, find creative solutions to our greatest challenges.

The stories I've told here are just a handful of the experiences that make up who I am as a forensic psychologist and a person. Hopefully they go some way to showing how everyone impacted by crime is unique. There really is no one kind of offender or victim. Each person comes with their own important stories to tell. It is possible to change the story though. Prevention is always better than a cure. By looking deeper at the root causes of extreme behaviour, we can start to write new beginnings.

Interview with the Author

Worldwide, almost 80 per cent of homicide victims are men, but in countless books, TV shows and films, extreme violence against women is the starting point of the story. Why do you think that is the case?

I call it the 'attractive women being hurt in interesting ways' trope. You are just as likely to find it in true crime books, documentaries and dramatizations as in the made-up-for-your-entertainment world. (It strikes me that 'true crime' is somewhat of a misnomer, as it is so skewed towards the re-telling of the most rare and appealing stories).Women, particularly young, beautiful, middle-class women, embody the 'ideal victim' that tends to resonate with audiences, a great percentage of whom are women themselves.

One theory is that women are attracted to these stories because what they are most afraid of is becoming the victim of violent crime themselves (yes, even us old, ugly ones). They feel that there is safety to be found in immersing themselves in the details of the worst possible scenarios. In that sense, stories about brutalized women are simultaneously anxiety-provoking and anxiety-relieving, which is an addictive combination.

As the interest in stories depicting violence against women has exploded, the portrayal of that violence has become more graphic, extreme and sexualized, I think largely for shock value in a crowded market. Put that together with glossy production values and glamorous actors and we are firmly in 'crime porn' territory.

What were your reasons for choosing the cases you talk about in the book? Was it a deliberate decision to focus on male homicide victims?

The cases chose themselves when I asked myself who, out of all of the hundreds of people I've come into contact with, had changed my thinking or direction in some way. For that reason, the book contains a number of career firsts: my first homicide case as an expert witness, my first time advising the police, and so on. I also wanted to include some stories, like those of Gary and Jeane, that wouldn't otherwise be told, despite being so representative of what goes on in criminal justice and mental health settings.

I didn't deliberately focus on telling stories involving men who have been killed. It just worked out that way. But I felt absolutely no need to include any additional cases involving female victims of homicide. It would have seemed gratuitous and I would rather chop off my writing hand than succumb to writing 'crime porn'.

Whether it's on the news or in the movies, why are we so fascinated by serial killers?

I'm not sure, as some of the serial killers I've met have been quite dull company.

We are social animals and we like to observe our fellow humans. The rise of reality television proves that we will watch people doing just about anything, but our brains are predisposed to pay specific attention to extreme and threatening behaviour. Serial killers speak to this primitive drive; they are as extreme and as threatening as one could imagine, after all, so best to keep a beady eye on them, despite the fact that we are more likely to be attacked by a cow than a serial killer.

Crime fiction is the UK's bestselling genre. Were you a reader of crime fiction before you became a forensic psychologist? Do you read it now?

I read a lot of true crime books in my teenage years but was less interested in fiction. I stopped reading anything crime-related at all, other than textbooks, as my career took off. I had enough real-world mayhem, with all of its traumatic ripple effects, to occupy my overworked brain without adding to it.

I've started to read some crime fiction just over the past twelve months. It turns out that I enjoy a good mystery as much as the next person (I'm most drawn to domestic noir) and at least I am guaranteed the satisfaction of a good resolution in the fictional world.

It does worry me, however, that the crime genre is so littered with misleading stereotypes – the super-intelligent serial killer, the dark-alley rapist, the psychotic loner – and throwaway collateral victims. It bothers me because the stories we tell, even the fictional ones, become internalized and inform people's beliefs about who criminals and victims are and how they 'should' behave. I see the consequences of these assumptions every day in my work, from juries reluctant to convict 'ordinary' men of rape and victims who don't come forward because they fear they won't be believed through to people with mental health problems who are shunned as being dangerous.

Maybe one day I'll have a go at writing some more nuanced and representative crime fiction myself. Not too representative though – the majority of crimes reported to police are property offences, and a book about a series of bicycle thefts might struggle to take off.

Knowing what you know now, what advice would you give your 21-year-old self?

Slow down! Notice more, question everything and ask for help. There is no need to be quite such a storm of ambition: no one, apart from yourself, expects you to pop up as a fully formed, hot-shot psychologist. It's fine to admit that you're still learning (you will always be learning). You do your best work when you are your most raw, curious and authentic self. Trust that one day – I can't pinpoint exactly when – you will wake up and be surprised to find that you actually are the person that you set out to be, and you won't care so much about what anybody else thinks of you.

There's a lot of dark humour in the book. Is humour a common coping mechanism in your line of work?

One of my all-time favourite quotes is from Carrie Fisher, who wrote: 'If my life wasn't funny it would just be true, and that is unacceptable.' She was talking about the therapeutic value of putting a comedic spin on even tragic or shocking events, and I couldn't agree more. I think that a gallows sense of humour is an essential and under-appreciated life skill. Poking fun at awful things is extremely common among emergency services personnel and also in mental health settings, from staff and patients alike. If, as a forensic psychologist, you don't naturally respond well to humour that is both a little bit wrong and a little bit right, I recommend you try to cultivate it, as this is one of your frontline tools for keeping a grip on your own resiliency and overall sanity, as well as that of others. Also, I have broken up more fights with improvised comedy routines than I could have hoped to if I had used only restraint techniques.

Dark humour comes very naturally to me, and for the book to be honest, that needed to be reflected in these pages. I do appreciate that to those who aren't familiar with the worlds in which I work, this type of humour might appear offhand or insensitive. As with all survival mechanisms, it has a time and a place, and I do try to be mindful of how I use it (especially in public).

Do you have any funny anecdotes that you can share?

I have many funny anecdotes that I would be best advised not to share! But a favourite moment comes from a client I mention briefly towards the end of the book. I first came across him when he was on a dirty protest in a local prison. He then popped up at various secure units I visited over the years, and the last time I saw him he was in a forensic step-down service, sixteen years after his original arrest, with only a week to go before moving to his own flat. He looked just like Freddie Mercury, complete with chevron moustache, and went around dressed in a Live Aid-era white vest and wristbands, even in the depths of winter. He bought a yellow cardigan and sewed gold epaulettes on to it. A couple of years after I first met him, he changed his name by deed poll – to Elton John.

Elton was on the autistic spectrum and, whenever I saw him, he used to tell me the same story, word for word. I loved hearing it and would often ask him to hold fire for a minute while I got myself a cup of tea and found somewhere comfy for us to sit, so I could really settle in and savour the full rendition of his tale. Although of course I never let him know quite how much I enjoyed it.

He had been a resident at a high-secure hospital where Dr Renton (the status-hungry supervisor I wrote about in Chapter 4) and Ian, a Welsh clinical psychologist with a magnificent vocabulary of swear words, both worked. It was well known that the pair despised each other. Elton described how these two men co-ran a therapy group and had once squared up to each other mid-session, in front of all their patients. Ian – the bigger person in everything but height – had punched Renton square in the face and given him a bloody nose, much to the amusement of their audience, who clapped and cheered ringside as the two grappled on the floor.

According to Elton, the group was Anger Management and this all took place next to a flipchart that asked 'When you are angry, where in your body do you feel it?'

You are an advocate for better conversations about mental health. Can you suggest some ways in which we can improve the way we talk about mental health?

I think it is fantastic that as a nation, we are being encouraged to talk more about our mental health and emotional wellbeing, but I do think that how we talk about them is significant. Increased awareness of mental health issues does have some unexpected downsides, one of which is the tendency to rush to declare an ever-expanding range of psychological events, such as grief, outbursts of anger or simply unpleasant behaviour or extreme political or religious views, as indicative of an illness or 'disorder'.

This really isn't helpful for many reasons. It is particularly annoying when people casually excuse their own poor behaviour by saying things like 'I'm a little bit bipolar' when what they really mean is 'I'm a little bit of a dickhead'. People who are grappling with genuine mental health problems have enough to deal with, without the negative associations certain labels can hold being perpetuated. Language is important and we can be more thoughtful in the way we use it.

The British Psychological Society advocates using ordinary language to describe a person's problems. Rather than saying that someone 'is a schizophrenic', it is more informative and less potentially disparaging to simply describe their experience: 'They are frightened because they hear threatening voices', for example. People deserve more than just being summed up in a single word, after all. This is an easy change that we can all make.

It is part of my job as a psychologist to help people make sense of the connections between their mental health struggles and the events, circumstances and relationships in their lives. But you don't have to be a psychologist to support friends or family members, you just need a willingness to listen to their stories in whatever words they want to use.

Reading Group Questions

Did you have any preconceived ideas about forensic psychology before reading *The Dark Side of the Mind*? Where did your information come from? Did reading this book make you see the work of a forensic psychologist differently?

How would you describe the culture of HMP Wakefield (Chapter 1) when Kerry Daynes started working there in 1996? What impact might this culture have had on the inmates and their rehabilitation? Where do cultures like this still exist today?

In Chapter 2, the author writes: 'Emotions need a voice. Without it they seep out eventually.' To what extent is Patrick a product of male socialization?

Why do you think Kerry Daynes chose to tell aspects of her own story alongside those of her clients?

Which story in this book stood out most for you and why? For example, did you find it disturbing, moving, sad or amusing?

How did you feel about the humour in the book?

If you were to find yourself in the unenviable position of being assessed by a forensic psychologist in a prison or secure unit, would you want them to be like Kerry Daynes in outlook?

Why do you think that Marcus (Chapter 5) was so reluctant to accept his diagnosis of schizophrenia? Do you think he should bear personal responsibility for killing his brother?

In the Epilogue, the author says that we cannot allow either empathy or anger to set the tone for how we respond to offenders. We must achieve 'rational compassion' instead. Which character in the book prompted the most feelings of empathy or anger?

In the Epilogue, the author says that 'our criminal justice system is not fit for purpose'. Do you agree? After reading this book, what kinds of changes would you like to see?

Notes & Further Reading

Chapter 1   Here Be Monsters

11   *Women make up 73 per cent*   Figures supplied by The British
Psychological Society, correct at August 2018

15   *It was the start of a mushrooming in prisoner numbers*   Commons
Library Briefing Paper CBP-04334, accessed online at https://
researchbriefings.files.parliament.uk/documents/SN04334/SN04334.
pdf on 23 July 2018. The Howard League provides a wealth of
statistics on the prison population at https://howardleague.org

22   *70 per cent of rape victims freeze*   Moller, A., Sondergaard, H.P. and
Helstrom, L., 2017, 'Tonic immobility during sexual assault – a
common reaction predicting post-traumatic stress disorder and
severe depression', *Acta Obstetricia et Gynecologia Scandinavica*, 96(8),
pp932-38

Chapter 2   Big Boys Don't Cry

35   *one of the highest prison suicide rates in Europe*   Fazel, S., Ramesh, T.
and Hawton, T., 2017, 'Suicide in prisons: an international study of
prevalence and contributory factors', *The Lancet Psychiatry*, 4(12),
pp946-52

36   *the Prison Reform Trust estimates 70 per cent*   Edgar, K. and Rickford,
D., 2009, 'Too Little, Too Late: An independent review of unmet
mental health need in prison', The Prison Reform Trust, accessed
online at www.prisonreformtrust.org.uk/Portals/0/Documents/
Too%20Little%20Too%20Late%20-%20a%20review%20of%20
unmet%20mental%20health%20need%20in%20prison%20.pdf

Chapter 3   The Blame Game

48 *95 per cent of our killers are male*   Gibbons, J., 2013, 'Global Study on Homicide', United Nations Office on Drugs and Crime, accessed online at www.unodc.org. See also Office for National Statistics, 2017, 'Homicide', accessed online at www.ons.gov.uk/peoplepopulationandcommunity/crimeandjustice/compendium/focusonviolentcrimeandsexualoffences/yearendingmarch2016/homicide

49 *Paul was in the approximate 10 per cent*   see also Karen Ingala Smith, 'Sex differences and Domestic Violence Murders', accessed online at https://kareningalasmith.com/counting-dead-women/ and Long, J., Harper, K. and Harvey, H., 2017, 'The Femicide Census: 2017 findings', accessed online at https://www.femicidecensus.org.uk

50 *domestic abuse is a gendered crime*   For instance, see Walby, S. and Towers, J., 2017, 'Measuring violence to end violence: mainstreaming gender', *Journal of Gender-Based Violence*, 1(1), pp11–31 and Myhill, A., 2017, 'Measuring domestic violence: context is everything', *Journal of Gender-Based Violence*, 1(1), pp33–44. Also see Office for National Statistics, 2018, 'Domestic abuse in England and Wales: Year ending March 2018', accessed online at www.ons.gov.uk/peoplepopulationandcommunity/crimeandjustice/bulletins/domesticabuseinenglandandwales/yearendingmarch2018

Chapter 4   Faking It

81 *Amy Cuddy*   2012, accessed online at www.ted.com/talks/amy_cuddy_your_body_language_shapes_who_you_are?language=en

96 *a classic experiment*   Rosenhan, D.L., 'On being sane in insane places', in Scheff, T.J. (ed.), *Labeling Madness*, Prentice-Hall (1975)

90 *normality is not 'real'* Caplan, Paula J., *They Say You're Crazy: How the world's most powerful psychiatrists decide who's normal*, Da Capo Press (1995)

Chapter 5 Witchdoctors and Brainwashers

108 *A 2012 study* Owen, P.R., 2012, 'Portrayals of schizophrenia by entertainment media: a content analysis of contemporary movies', *Psychiatric Services,* 63(7), pp655–9

109 *50 and 70 cases* see 'Violence and mental health: the facts', 2019, Time To Change, accessed at www.time-to-change.org.uk/media-centre/responsible-reporting/violence-mental-health-problems

109 *Research tells us* For a critical review see 'Risk distortion and risk assessment', in Sidley, G., *Tales From The Madhouse*, PCCS Books (2015)

111 *effectiveness in preventing reoffending* For instance, see Falshaw, L. et al., 2003, 'Searching for "What Works": an evaluation of cognitive skills programmes'. Home Office Research, Findings 206. For a critique see Forde, Robert A., *Bad Psychology: How forensic psychology left science behind*, Jessica Kingsley Publishers (2018)

112 *Bennett Inquiry* Report accessed at http://image.guardian.co.uk/sys-files/Society/documents/2004/02/12/Bennett.pdf

113 *mental health services are riddled with racial discrimination* For instance, see Equality and Human Rights Commission (EHRC), October 2018, 'Is Britain Fairer?', accessed online at www.equalityhumanrights.com/en/publication-download/britain-fairer-2018. See also Servicegovuk, 2019, accessed online at www.ethnicity-facts-figures.service.gov.uk/health/access-to-treatment/detentions-under-the-mental-health-act/latest

119 *Dr Jay Watts* 'Mental health labels can save lives. But they can also destroy them', *Guardian*, 24 April 2018

119 *mental distress is more likely a product of complex, overlapping personal and social factors* See Kinderman, P., *The New Laws of Psychology: Why nature and nurture alone can't explain human behaviour*, Constable & Robinson (2014). More information can be also be found at www.madintheuk.com and www.adisorder4everyone.com

121 *83 per cent described* Millham, A. and Easton, S., 1998, 'Prevalence of auditory hallucinations in nurses in mental health', *Journal of Psychiatric and Mental Health Nursing*, 5, pp95–9

Chapter 6   Power Plays

132 *UK criminologists estimate* Gresswell, D.M. and Hollin, C.R., 1994, 'Multiple murder: a review', *British Journal of Criminology*, 34, pp1–14

132 *it has blossomed into its own distinct discipline* For a detailed overview, I recommend Canter, D. and Youngs, D., *Investigative Psychology: Offender profiling and the analysis of criminal action*, John Wiley & Sons (2009)

135 *the majority of break-ins to homes* Office for National Statistics, 2017, 'Overview of burglary and other household theft: England and Wales', accessed online at www.ons. gov.uk/peoplepopulationandcommunity/crimeandjustice/ articles/overviewofburglaryandotherhouseholdtheft/ englandandwales#what-are-the-long-term-trends

155 *US lie detection expert* See Ekman, P., *Telling Lies*, W.W. Norton & Company (2009)

155 *the 3-2-7 rule* Archer, D.E. and Lansley, C.A., 2015, 'Public

appeals, news interviews and crocodile tears: an argument for multi-channel analysis', accessed online at www.euppublishing.com

Chapter 7 Insults and Injuries

161 *we can predict statistically* Forde, Robert A., *Bad Psychology: How Forensic Psychology Left Science Behind,* Jessica Kingsley Publishers (2018)

167 *the latest Crime Survey for England and Wales* Office for National Statistics, 2018, 'Sexual offences in England and Wales: year ending March 2017', accessed online at www.ons.gov. uk/peoplepopulationandcommunity/crimeandjustice/articles/ sexualoffencesinenglandandwales/yearendingmarch2017

179 *proportion of people with brain injuries* Williams, W.H. et al., 2018, 'Traumatic brain injury: a potential cause of violent crime', *The Lancet Psychiatry*, 5(10), pp836-844

179 *around 30 per cent... People aged 60 or over* Hewson, A., 2018, 'Bromley Briefings Prison Factfile Autumn 2018', The Prison Reform Trust, accessed online at www.prisonreformtrust.org. uk/Portals/0/Documents/Bromley%20Briefings/Autumn%20 2018%20Factfile.pdf

Chapter 8 A Man's World

188 *A 2017 study* Amnesty International, 2018, 'Online abuse of women is widespread in UK'. accessed online at www.amnesty. org/en/latest/news/2018/12/crowdsourced-twitter-study-reveals- shocking-scale-of-online-abuse-against-women/

190 *one in five* See *Homicides, Firearm offences and intimate violence 2009/10; Supplementary Volume 2 to Crime in England and Wales*

2009/10, 2nd Edition, Home Office Statistical Bulletin 01/11

194 *94 per cent*   Monckton-Smith, J., Szymanska, K. and Haile, S., 2017, 'Exploring the Relationship between Stalking and Homicide', Suzy Lamplugh Trust, accessed online at http://eprints.glos.ac.uk/4553/

195 *likely to escalate into violence*   Mullen, P., Pathe, M. and Purcell, R., *Stalkers and Their Victims*, Cambridge University Press (2009)

196 *just because you're paranoid*   Heller, Joseph, *Catch 22*, Vintage (1955)

198 *The Stalking Risk Profile*   see www.stalkingriskprofile.com

198 *'The Psychopath Test'*   Ronson, J., *The Psychopath Test*, Picador (2011)

201 *The Psychopathy Checklist*   See Hart, S.D., Hare, R.D., and Harpur, T.J., 'The Psychopathy Checklist – Revised (PCL – R): An overview for researchers and clinicians', in J.C. Rosen and P. McReynolds (eds), *Advances in Psychological Assessment*, Vol. 8, pp103-30, Plenum Press (1992). As an overview for the general reader, see Hare, R., *Without Conscience*, Guilford Press (1999)

202 *the PCL-R is also the subject of much debate*   For instance, see Skeem et al., 2011, 'Psychopathic personality: bridging the gap between scientific evidence and public policy', *Psychological Science in the Public Interest*, 12(3), pp95-162. For an accessible discussion of the issues for the general reader, see Forde, R.A., *Bad Psychology: how forensic psychology left science behind,* Jessica Kingsley Publishers (2018)

202 *one 2016 study*   Brooks, N. and Frizon, K., 2016, 'Psychopathic personality characteristics among high functioning populations', *Crime Psychology Review*, 2(1), pp22-44

207 *my favourite research study*   Cooke et al., 2005, 'Assessing psychopathy in the UK: concerns about cross-cultural generalisability', *British Journal of Psychiatry*, 186, pp339-45

Chapter 9   The Case of the Missing Finger

222   *The National Crime Agency estimates*   *Independent*, 3 September 2018, accessed online at www.independent.co.uk/news/uk/home-news/uk-online-sex-threat-80000-people-children-national-crime-agency-a8519606.html

227   *42 per cent according to a report*   Newiss, G., 2013, 'Taken: A study of child abduction in the UK. Parents and Abducted Children Together (PACT) and the Child Exploitation and Online Protection Centre (CEOP)', accessed online at www.actionagainstabduction.org/wp-content/uploads/2015/02/Taken.pdf

Chapter 10   Safe and Sound

243   *there is a certain unsavoury pleasure*   Tallis, Frank, *The Incurable Romantic: and other unsettling revelations*, Little, Brown (2018)

Chapter 11   The Sum of Our Parts

264   *dissociative identity disorder*   For information and support with dissociative experiences and information for professionals, see PODS (Positive Outcomes for Dissociative Survivors), www.pods-online.org.uk

Epilogue

281   *National Centre for Domestic Violence*   www.ncdv.org.uk. Referrals can be made online or by telephone: 0207 186 8270

281   *Suzy Lamplugh Trust*   www.suzylamplugh.org, National Stalking Helpline: 0808 802 0300

284   Bloom, P., *Against Empathy: The case for rational compassion*,   Vintage (2016)

Acknowledgements

First and foremost, I must thank Sarah Thompson for walking with me throughout the writing of this memoir. I hope that, in time, you will be welcome again in the numerous coffee shops I embarrassed you in. In addition, I couldn't have got to the finishing line without the advice, input and general cheerleading of Daniel Coleman-Cooke.

The Dark Side of the Mind would not have been written if it were not for Sylvia Tidy-Harris (and Fredders) at Tidy Management. You are more than just a great agent, you are also the best of people and I'm so pleased to have found you. My appreciation also goes to Jonathan Conway at the Jonathan Conway Literary Agency and to Claudia Connal and the entire, excellent team at Octopus. Thank you for seeing the potential in my stories, I am truly honoured to carry the Endeavour logo on this book.

Special thanks to Susan Bradley for your above-and-beyond 'general reader' feedback on early drafts of the book. At times it was hard to take and fear I may see shocked Beaker memes in my nightmares for years to come, but your tough love, counsel and encouragement spurred me on.

To Gary Sidley, many thanks for your supervision of the language used in this book and supportive prods to keep writing throughout the process. Also to Jo Watson at Drop The Disorder for the introduction. Your thought-provoking questioning of the culture of psychiatry resonates deeply with me, I will gladly join your revolution.

ACKNOWLEDGEMENTS

To Kate in the little cafe in the park where I walk my dogs, this book has been fuelled by your tea, cheese and onion toasties and Ugg therapy. A friendly, safe space with a huge amount of community spirit makes more of a difference to people than you know. As I am a vegetarian, the bacon scraps make more of a difference to Fozzchops and Humphrey than you might imagine too.

My thanks and respect to the various colleagues I have worked alongside over the years who, despite facing daily challenges, limited resources and a lack of acknowledgement of their worth, have maintained their humour, compassion and enthusiasm to make a positive impact – you know who you are.

And finally, to my family, who I worry half to death. Annoying as it is to admit it, the three of you are written into every page of this book, because you are written into me, and I couldn't feel more grateful for you.

About the Author

Kerry Daynes is a consultant forensic psychologist. She is often invited to act as psychological specialist in major police investigations and is a trusted advisor to the British government regarding the safe management of high-risk individuals. Kerry is a sought-after speaker and provides regular commentary for international television networks. She is an advocate for better conversations on mental health and is a patron of the National Centre for Domestic Violence and Talking2Minds.

www.kerrydaynes.online